Sensory Integration.................................................. 189
*Touch* .................................................................. 190
*Movement*............................................................. 190
*Body Position*........................................................ 190
*Sight* ................................................................... 191
*Sound* .................................................................. 191
*Smell*.................................................................... 191
*Taste*.................................................................... 191
Alternative Therapies ............................................ 192
Nutrition................................................................ 193
ALCOHOLISM ....................................................... 197
Sugar and the Recovering Alcoholic ..................... 204
WEIGHT LOSS ....................................................... 206
DEPRESSION ......................................................... 212
ANXIETY ............................................................... 214
SINUSES................................................................. 216
Nutritional Support and Other Considerations for
Sinus (and Other) Infections .................................. 220
ASTHMA................................................................. 223
OTHER HEALTH PROBLEMS................................ 226
NOW WHAT? ......................................................... 227
CONCLUSION........................................................ 229
APPENDIX: RECIPES ............................................. 233

## PREFACE

This book is written for people who are going to the office of someone trained in nutrition. If you are seeking the help of a chiropractor, naturopath, nutritionist or other professional, it can help you to understand a little about nutrition and the natural approach to health. It can help you to understand what your health care provider is trying to do for you. Unfortunately, information about health makes treating yourself tempting.

Most people would not dream of replacing their car's transmission by themselves without training, yet have no problem trying to treat their own health problems or to overrule the decisions made by their health care provider. Most patients follow advice pretty well, but there are some patients who do not. They can be told to come back in a week, but manage to decide that two or three weeks would be better. They modify their treatment based on articles read in the popular press and frequently manage to find advice that they follow like Charlton Heston handed it to them on a stone tablet, even though they already go to a trained professional.

A book like this often compounds the practitioner's problems by being the unseen "expert" against which all of the practitioner's decisions are judged. I have this problem in my own office. There is an absolutist nature to most self-help books that make the reader absolutely believe what is written. For example, I tend to let patients with Candidiasis eat some fruit. Often a patient will read a book that tells them not to eat fruit. It will tell them not to eat fruit for 40 pages with the vehemence of an eighteenth century Calvinist preacher. Woe unto those who eat fruit, etc. The patient will then come into the office with his newfound fear of fruit, looking at me like I just knocked Charlton Heston down and took away his stone tablets.

Everyone doing nutritional counseling has also had the experience of having his or her therapy second-guessed by some guy working in a health food store. There was one woman in particular, who was actually doing pretty well with the advice she was getting, came into the office and said, "How come you didn't tell me I needed Bee pollen?" after a trip to the health food store. The point is to find someone whose expertise you respect and follow his or her advice and don't second-guess the advice, even if the advice is a little different than what you read here.

The thing about natural health care is that many things work, and it is as much art as it is science. Many different approaches work. After 20 years of practice, I still talk to doctors who teach me new (and often better) ways of doing things. No one has all of the answers, and beware of people who tell you that they do.

As a practitioner I have a love/hate relationship with popular books on health. It is easy to appreciate what a book has to say and to find value in it without agreeing with everything in the book. For example, I frequently recommend *Sugar Busters* to patients. It presents a very effective way to lose weight for people who are not ready for stricter, healthier programs. So very many Americans are insulin insensitive, and refined carbohydrates are the source of their weight problem. It is a less extreme diet than the Atkins diet, with similar results. But *Sugar Busters* does recommend nitrated meats and does not do a good job telling people to avoid chemicals and hydrogenated oils. Also, there are issues that it doesn't address, issues like food allergies or alkaline/acid balance. However, it still is a pretty good diet to give someone, who in the past, has paid no attention to food quality and who has trouble losing weight.

This book does make specific product recommendations. Biotics Research is mentioned by name throughout the book. I do use other products. (I discussed this with the folks at Biotics. There were some tears and some hugs, but we finally decided that I could see other vitamin companies and they could see other doctors.) At first I had a problem with commercializing the book in this way, but it really isn't much different from the relationship between doctors, medical journals and drug companies.

Drug companies link themselves to doctors' education in a very big way. They endow the medical schools, they sponsor postgraduate education and they buy advertisements in the medical journals. They have positioned themselves to completely influence the medical profession. Eisenhower coined the phrase "military industrial complex" to describe the interrelationship between the Pentagon and the defense industry. We also have a "medical pharmaceutical complex." Is it any wonder that there is so little research to support natural health care? If you are making $3 billion per year selling antidepressants, would you keep your ad in a journal that published an article about folic acid helping with depression? Actually the influence goes beyond single bits of research. The drug companies influence the medical schools, postgraduate education for doctors and the journals. The drug companies really influence medicines paradigm—how doctors think about health and disease.

With this in mind, Biotics Research products are endorsed in this book. Just as the medical profession and the drug companies support each other, we in natural health care need to do the same. We are smaller both financially and politically. Every so often we have to fight in Congress to keep the right to buy supplements. There is a prejudice against supplements in the government. For years, many people used tryptophan as a safe, natural way to help control depression and to help them sleep. The FDA has banned tryptophan, simply because a bad batch made some people sick. A similar action to this would be to ban milk because of a salmonella outbreak.

So I have no trouble supporting a company that supports natural health care and my profession. Biotics Research Corporation is family-owned and extremely accessible to practitioners. Doctors can tour the plant and see the company's quality control. It is impressive. Biotics Research is also innovative: the company is constantly in contact with doctors in the field learning what works for these doctors and helping them develop new and better products.

There are other companies that I would happily write an endorsement for, others that I would not. I would not recommend a company that had shoddy quality control or whose products do not meet label claims any more than I would do a cigarette ad. So, yes there is a little bit of a commercial for Biotics Research here, but they are good folks and have done a lot to advance the cause of natural health care. If your health care provider recommends different products, trust that he or she has looked into the quality control issue and has your best interests at heart. We all do things a little differently.

## INTRODUCTION

One of my nightmares is where I receive a letter from the law offices of McGreedy, Larsen and Snatch. The letter states that their client, a Mr. I. M. Needlebrain read one of my books and pursued a course of self-treatment. It goes on to say that the unfortunate Mr. Needlebrain had been suffering from a case of Fecalith Systematica, and had he sought out *proper* medical assistance, he could have been easily cured with a course of antibiotics and an enema.

The letter goes on to say that reading the book convinced Mr. Needlebrain that he could treat himself. The fact that the book did not advise him of the possibility that he had Fecalith Systematica constitutes negligence. As a result, he wasted valuable time trying *questionable* treatments, while his health continued to decline. His health became worse, and he finally went into a coma and is not expected to live. His estranged family, overcome with grief, is suing for *$50* million, my *Mad* magazine collection and my firstborn child.

The point is, don't try to be your own doctor. I don't have $50 million dollars, my mother burned my *Mad* magazine collection in 1976 and my firstborn is quite a handful. (Besides she'd be about 43 by the time all of the court proceedings were over.)

Fatigue is a symptom that is present in many serious diseases including cancer, diabetes and AIDS. No book can anticipate every possible health problem or be a substitute for proper health care. It can, however, help you to make healthier choices.

The amount of energy you have is proportional to how healthy you are. Being healthy is not just a matter of not being sick. Health is when all of the body's organs and systems are functioning optimally. If the organs and systems of your body are not working at their best, you become fatigued.

Proper nutrition, activity, waste removal, rest and genetics are all vital to optimum health. If these components are not supplied, the body begins a progression that ends in disease.

Poor nutrition, inactivity, improper waste removal and lack of rest do not immediately cause health problems. However, when denied the necessary components of health, individual cells begin to function poorly. Health is less than optimal, but there are no symptoms—at least at first.

Dr. Emanuel Cheraskin created the following model for poor health. Poor health is usually the result of the following progression: ***Bad habits, lack of necessary components of health*** $\rightarrow$ ***poor cell function*** $\rightarrow$ ***poor enzyme function*** $\rightarrow$ ***poor endocrine function*** $\rightarrow$ ***poor immune system function*** $\rightarrow$ ***malaise*** $\rightarrow$ ***symptoms*** $\rightarrow$ ***signs, or diagnosable disease.***

Alan Gaby, MD, had a very clever way of describing a descent into poor health. He said that it was a progression that went: "Big Mac, Zantac, Prozac." In other words, you eat crap, your digestion goes so you take a drug that further hinders digestion and nutrient absorption, and then you start having problems with depression. Disease progresses from poor habits.

You never hear someone say, "Yesterday I came down with cancer." Chronic disease does not just happen all of a sudden. It evolves after a departure from ideal health.

Even infectious disease needs a relatively unhealthy body to find a home. The bubonic plague killed half of the people in Europe in the fourteenth century. That means the other half didn't get the disease; they were healthier.

We say things like, "Yesterday I caught a cold." That implies that everyone around you "missed" the cold. The germs, with Michael Jordan-like moves, faked right, spun left, avoiding everyone else and slam-dunked into you. At work, school or any place where a lot of people are together, there are people who are sick all of the time and there are people who are never sick. Do the germs keep missing the same people all of the time? Of course not. People who don't get sick have better cell function, enzyme function, hormone function, immune system function and better overall health. Modern medicine is sickness oriented and most people suffering from fatigue are not sick. They just aren't very healthy.

Wouldn't it be wise to treat your health before you developed a disease? If your car runs reasonably well and you take it to a mechanic, he doesn't say, "There's nothing wrong with your car, bring it to me when it doesn't run." A car has need of a mechanic, even when it is running. It needs regular maintenance to keep it running. The mechanic will change the oil and spark plugs in an otherwise "healthy" car. He doesn't wait until the engine locks up from lack of oil.

We live in a time of skyrocketing medical costs. When it is discussed on the news, it is always called "health care." Medical intervention, after a lifetime of ignoring health, is expensive, but it isn't health care; it's sickness care. Sickness care is expensive; health care is actually pretty inexpensive. Isn't it wiser to begin to return to ideal health than it is to wait until you have a disease that your doctor can name and give you a drug or other medical treatment?

We tend to want to abuse our bodies for a lifetime, and when we start having problems, we want to go to a doctor and have it fixed (preferably without any inconvenience or pain). A lot of the health care dollar is spent on new technology and extensive treatment for serious diseases. Very little is spent on prevention or education.

Many people come into the offices of health care practitioners complaining about fatigue, skin problems, sinusitis, digestive disorders and other

10

chronic problems. Few see the connection between their lifestyle and how they feel.

Alice (not her real name—it's actually Janet) was an artist who not only suffered from fatigue, but also had a horrible skin rash on her hands. It had gotten so bad that the skin was peeling off. They cracked, bled and were very painful. She had been to an internist, an allergist and a dermatologist and was unable to get a satisfactory diagnosis or an effective treatment. Combined, her doctors had close to 30 years of education among them. She was being treated with a steroid ointment that didn't seem to do her much good.

When she came into the office she was told to write down all of the food she consumed for one week. A typical day's food for her was as follows: Eight cups of coffee, butterscotch pudding and a pork chop, and that was a good day. She ate only one meal per day. She ate no fruits or vegetables. She drank no water, only coffee.

I convinced her to change her diet. She was motivated because her hands had gotten so bad that she couldn't work. After a few weeks of proper eating and some vitamin supplementation, her rash was almost completely healed.

The cure was so simple that it was laughable that she had so much trouble getting help. She only needed someone to treat the patient who had the rash and not simply treat the rash.

Her doctors looked at the rash, compared it to other rashes they had seen and gave her the drug that usually worked for rashes. The problem wasn't that her doctors weren't skilled or dedicated. The problem was one of philosophy. Thinking of an illness as an enemy to be destroyed is often not as effective as helping the body return to normal physiology.

How expensive was it for her to see an internist and two specialists, have tests and fill prescriptions? The cost of her sickness care was much more than the cost of what returned her to health, a simple change in her diet. Doctors' visits, tests and drugs are much more expensive than water, vegetables and other healthy food. Sickness care is much more expensive than health care.

## YOUR HABITS AFFECT HOW YOU FEEL

If your car doesn't start or run well, the first thing you do is to make sure that it has gas and that the battery is charged. You put in new spark plugs or make sure that the fuel filter is clean. You don't immediately overhaul the engine. You check for small, common things that are easily repaired. Similarly, small changes in your day-to-day habits will give you more energy than you thought possible. Supplying your body with its basic needs will ensure good health. Being healthy means having plenty of energy.

Just as a car needs gas, oil, electricity and occasional cleaning and replacement of components, the body needs oxygen, nutrients, proper elimination of waste, structural stability and movement. Unfortunately, most of us take better care of our cars than we do our bodies.

Your body is made up of billions of cells. Each cell is like a tiny factory that needs oxygen, nutrients and water and needs to eliminate waste in order to continue to function and produce its products. If your cells are healthy, you are healthy. If you are healthy, you have plenty of energy.

### Breathing

Denying your body oxygen will kill it faster than denying it anything else. You can live for weeks without food, for days without water, but only for minutes without oxygen. We all take breathing for granted, but it is the most important thing we do. It defines life.

Yoga and various martial arts recognize the importance of breathing. In Yoga there are a variety of breathing exercises, such as the cleansing breath or the breath of fire. In Yoga, Pranayama is the rhythmic control of breath. According to the book, *Light on Pranayama* by B.K.S. Iyengar, during normal inhalation, an average person takes in about 500 cubic centimeters of air. During deep inhalation, the volume is six times as great. The Yogis believed that deep breathing energizes the body and cleanses the nadis, which are organs of the "subtle" body. In other words, there are not only physical and mental benefits to deep breathing, but also spiritual benefits.

Most of us breathe too shallowly and do not get good oxygenation of our tissues with each breath. Deep breathing can, at the same time, relax you and energize you. Try it now. Exhale and force all of the air out of your lungs. Slowly, deeply breathe the air back in. Use your diaphragm and fill your lungs to capacity. Pause for a few seconds with your lungs full. Exhale, even more slowly than you inhaled; take twice as long to exhale as you did to inhale. Force all of the air out of your lungs. Slowly inhale again and repeat the process. Do this for 10 breaths.

Notice the difference in how you feel after doing the deep breathing. If you didn't do the exercise, please do it now. It will make a difference in how you feel, and it will demonstrate to you just how much deep breathing can energize you. Deep breathing does two things. It delivers oxygen to the tissues and it increases lymphatic circulation.

Lymph is fluid that seeps from the capillaries and bathes all of the cells. The lymphatic system is sort of a storm sewer for the blood stream and is also a key part of the immune system. It removes waste products from the cells like a storm sewer, gathering runoff from the bloodstream and wastes from the cells. It is also one of the major routes for absorption of nutrients from the digestive system. If lymphatic flow is sluggish, your body's cells sit in their own waste. The cells also do not receive sufficient oxygen or nutrients.

Deep breathing increases the lymphatic flow. When you breathe deeply, you get oxygen to your cells and you help them to remove waste. The effects are felt almost immediately.

## Water

The adult human body is about 56% fluid. Individual cells contain between 70% and 85% water. Water is necessary for proper elimination of wastes and for good lymphatic flow.

Many people think that the body produces urine to get rid of excess water. Actually, the body produces urine in order to get rid of small amounts of solid waste. It uses water, which is precious to it, to get rid of these wastes.

When patients are told to drink eight, eight-ounce glasses of water each day, they usually say, "If I drank that much water, I'd live in the bathroom." If this is you, it means that you really need the water. Your body is holding onto waste products, waiting for you to have enough sense to drink water so it can get rid of the wastes.

Recently a study was published that stated that people were being told to drink too much water, and that too much water could be harmful. Actually, if the subjects of the study only drank water, six or eight glasses per day would not be a problem. The trouble is that too many people drink diuretics like coffee and colas. They drink sugared, flavored drinks, or worse, drinks with artificial sweeteners. These things are the problem, not the water.

Inadequate water intake decreases the lymphatic circulation, causing poor tissue oxygenation and waste removal. Waste products that should be carried away from the cell by the lymphatic system stay in the vicinity of the cell. You sit there marinating in your own waste products. Of course you're fatigued.

One of the main causes of constipation is inadequate water consumption. The large intestine is the final five feet of the digestive tract. It produces no enzymes and absorbs few nutrients. The one thing that is absorbed in the large intestine is water. If a person is not properly hydrated, more water is absorbed from the large intestine than would be if the person drank plenty of water. This makes the stool dry and hard, resulting in constipation.

Constipation causes fatigue. The intestinal lymph nodes of someone suffering from chronic constipation are full of bacteria. This can contribute to leaky gut, dysbiosis and to immune system problems, all of which contribute to fatigue and even more serious health problems. People who are chronically constipated have a better chance of getting colon cancer.

People with constipation often take fiber. Fiber increases the bulk of the stool and stimulates the digestive tract to move faster. If the individual taking the fiber needs water, the stool becomes dry and hard and is not easily eliminated. It's a paradox: taking fiber laxatives can actually make constipation worse. Very often increasing water intake "cures" constipation where taking fiber does not.

Fiber is also important if you want to bring constipation under control, but it is best to get your fiber from eating plenty of fresh fruits and vegetables, not fiber supplements. Simply drinking water and eating fruits and vegetables cures most cases of constipation. If it does not, then there may be a problem with dysbiosis, hydrochloric acid, enzymes, the thyroid or there may be a need for bile salts. These topics will be covered later.

Water quality is an important issue. The Environmental Protection Agency (EPA) has warned that the water in many areas is not fit to drink. If water quality is bad enough for the government to notice, it must be pretty bad. In 1995 people became sick in Milwaukee from bacteria that was not removed from their municipal water supply. Lead from old pipes often finds its way into tap water. This has been a big problem in the Chicago area. Drinking tap water may not be a good idea. Your health care provider can help you decide which source of water is best.

There is a lot of controversy about what kind of water is best. Spring water is very rich in minerals, especially iron and calcium. Unfortunately, much of the water is polluted with pesticides and industrial waste. Every so often you hear about an inordinate number of people, living in the same area, dying of cancer. Chemicals in the water supply may be one possible explanation of this.

There are labs that will test your water for various pollutants. Testing and filtering tap water is a good idea. City tap water has a lot of chlorine and fluorine in it. Even the government says not all tap water is safe. In some areas there is lead in the drinking water. There are kits you can buy to test the water yourself. National Testing Lab, Inc. in Cleveland, Ohio will test your water for heavy metals, pesticides and other contaminants for a modest fee. The lab's phone number is 800-458-3330.

Water quality is important, but don't let worrying about your water keep you from drinking enough of it. Not consuming enough water can cause fatigue, constipation and even sinus trouble.

## GENERAL NUTRITION

### Vitamins

Vitamins are frequently recommended in health food stores to people who suffer from fatigue. Convenience stores sell "energy packs" consisting of three or four different vitamins, promising to give whoever takes them more energy.

Patients frequently ask what vitamin is good for fatigue. Taking vitamins, however, does not guarantee you more energy. In order for a vitamin to do you any good, you must need it.

You don't take a vitamin to make a specific physiologic change, like you would take a drug. Nutrients are effective in treating illness because many of the symptoms people suffer with are the result of nutrient deficiency. People try to use them like drugs—addressing specific symptoms. Patients are continually saying things like, "I heard vitamin E will help my virility," or "I heard that vitamin B will give me more energy." Using vitamins to address specific symptoms doesn't always work. If your fatigue is caused by a B vitamin deficiency, taking B vitamins will increase your energy. If you are deficient in vitamin E, taking vitamin E may increase your virility. We commonly hear doctors say the vitamins can't cure disease and in a sense they are right, with one important exception. Vitamins cure the disease of vitamin deficiency. So while it looks like vitamins and minerals are "curing" a health problem, what is really happening is the nutrient is enabling the body to function normally. Keeping that in mind, here are some examples of problems caused by nutritional deficiency:

*Vitamin $B_6$ deficiency* can cause you to react unfavorably to MSG (Chinese restaurant syndrome).

*Molybdenum deficiency* may cause you to be sensitive to smoke and perfume.

*Deficiencies of folic acid or $B_{12}$* can be a source of infertility.

*Deficiency of $B_{12}$* can cause memory problems and even dementia in older people—sometimes symptoms are so severe that it is mistaken for Alzeheimer's disease.

*Zinc deficiency* can cause immune system problems, sugar cravings or skin problems.

*Magnesium deficiency* can cause muscle spasms or heart arrythmias. Asthmatics frequently improve with magnesium supplementation. Women who have breast tenderness and mood swings during their menstrual cycle need magnesium.

*Essential fatty acid deficiency* can cause skin problems, muscle fatigue or tension headaches.

*Vitamin B complex deficiencies* can cause fatigue or depression.

*Folic acid deficiency* can cause depression, anemia and a low white cell count.

*Anemias that don't respond to iron* supplementation may indicate a need of folic acid, $B_{12}$, vitamin A, protein, copper or hydrochloric acid.

*Deficiencies in magnesium, calcium or essential fatty acids* can be a source of menstrual cramps.

*Adequate selenium* is necessary to effectively fight a viral infection.

*Vitamin A deficiency* can cause vision, immune system or skin problems. Also, Hay fever sufferers with itchy eyes are frequently deficient in vitamin A.

These are just some of the problems caused by nutritional deficiency. There are many others. For example, people with many allergies are commonly deficient in trace minerals. People who get chronic headaches frequently improve when supplemented with magnesium. Virtually every function in the human body—including thought—is the result of a biochemical reaction. Good nutrition ensures good biochemical function. Not all immune system problems are caused by zinc deficiency and not all muscle spasms are the result of magnesium deficiency. This is the reason than one person can begin to take zinc and stop having colds and another takes zinc with seemingly no benefit. Zinc fixes a zinc deficiency, not the immune system (unless the immune problem is caused by the zinc deficiency). You need to stop thinking of vitamins and minerals in terms of treatment and more in terms of correcting a deficiency.

## Taking Supplements

Having a health care professional who is trained in nutrition is much better than trying to treat yourself according to your symptoms. You wouldn't treat yourself with drugs; you would seek the help of a professional, a doctor. So should it be with nutrition.

Taking nutrients without the advice of a professional may be safer than self-medicating with drugs, but if you want good results, seek professional advice. Biochemistry and nutrition are complicated subjects. You don't know what you don't know until you know what you didn't know. So many people are taking herbs and nutrients without knowing or understanding what they are taking.

Another reason to seek professional advice is the quality of the products available to professionals. Someone who deals with nutritional and herbal products is more likely to know which companies have good quality control and which formulas are likely to work. There is not a lot of quality control in the food supplement industry and we pretty much have to trust the companies we deal with. A company like Biotics Research has excellent quality control. It produces supplements to pharmacological standards. It is also innovative. Take something simple, like tableting base. Most companies use inert material. Some even use talc. Biotics makes its tableting agent part of the nutrient. It is a vegetable culture and it has phytochemical and antioxidant activity all by itself, before any nutrient is added. It is very well absorbed and utilized by the body. The body actually treats it like food. You will not find vitamins of this quality in your local drug store.

If there is a need for a particular vitamin, or an extreme deficiency, taking that vitamin will create what seems like a miracle. One person will take a vitamin B complex and become energetic. Another will take it and feel no effects at all. The first person needed vitamin B; the second did not. A vitamin is not effective unless there is a deficiency, even a slight one. If you are tired, and you need vitamin B, it will help you. If your fatigue is due to something else, you can take a pound of vitamin B and it won't make any difference.

Because of mechanized agriculture, produce is often lacking in trace nutrients. A lifetime of poor eating habits, chemical exposure, drug therapies and other assaults on the body makes vitamin supplementation necessary. Taking vitamins like they're drugs to target ailments is not always an effective strategy. Supplementation is just what the word implies: you augment a diet of nutrient-rich foods. Most of your vitamins should be gotten from good food; you *supplement* to help yourself in deficient areas. Some people are deficient in a lot of nutrients, and will benefit by taking lots of different vitamins. Others will find that a diet of whole foods supplies them with all of the vitamins and minerals they need.

It is true that someone fighting a cold may benefit from vitamin C, someone under stress may benefit from vitamin B, and someone with libido problems may benefit from vitamin E. People suffering from allergies and extreme fatigue have been helped by taking large doses of nutrients. However, nutritional therapy is not like drug therapy. There is an interrelationship among nutrients. Balance is as important, if not more important, than absolute amounts. In fact, taking too much of the wrong vitamin may aggravate your problem. Skill and an understanding of physiology and nutrition are needed to effectively use nutritional supplementation to improve your health.

Let's say, for example, that you tend to have bladder infections. You read that vitamin C is good for immune system problems and infections and you take large doses of it. If you are vitamin A deficient (which may cause the membrane of the bladder to be more susceptible to infection), and if your urine tends to be acidic, taking large doses of vitamin C may not help you.

Which vitamin will help with fatigue? The answer is simple: the one you are most deficient in. Nutrition and physiology are very complex. There are thousands of biochemical reactions going on in the body all of the time. Vitamins and minerals make these reactions possible. Even slight deficiencies in nutrients can affect the body's biochemistry. Often nothing is medically wrong, except for fatigue or another vague symptom.

You may notice Ed in accounting. He's the guy who used to shuffle through the office, head down, eyes at half-mast. Suddenly Ed seems to have a new lease on life. He takes up squash, bungi jumping and mountain climbing, and gets a 19-year-old girlfriend. You're impressed because Ed is 96 (and he doesn't even use Armor-all on his dashboard). You ask him his secret and he shows you his new stress vitamin that is packed with antioxidants, ginseng, bee pollen, Chinese herbs and some kind of extract made from hummingbird testicles. Ed tells you all of this at his villa in Hawaii, during a recruitment meeting for a multilevel marketing plan to sell this vitamin. He got in early, at the top of the pyramid, so he earns more than the gross national product of several small countries. You figure that you could use a little more energy and the money sounds good, so you try it. You begin by investing $600 for some of the product and the basic sales kit. After you start taking the supplement you get sick to your stomach and break out in purple spots. Ed says not to worry; it's just part of the detox. You become a little concerned when the detox lasts for three and a half years. Your spots don't go away, and in three and a half years you've only managed to sell two bottles of the stuff. (The purple spots are a real deterrent to sales.) It just doesn't work.

If the guy at the health food store, the article in *Prevention* magazine or Ed picks a vitamin that you are deficient in, and you try it, you'll feel better. If it doesn't have anything you need, it won't do you much good. Ed's body needed extract of hummingbird testicles, and yours didn't.

Even if you take a vitamin that your body needs, this does not guarantee that you'll feel better. You may have health issues that override the small improvement that taking a necessary vitamin may provide. You may read an article that tells you that vitamin B complex reduces stress and increases energy. You may realize that you are vitamin B deficient because you know that you eat a lot of sugar and starch. Your diet and stress level created a need for B vitamins, but if you have a lot of other health problems, you may not notice any improvement from taking the B vitamins.

## Maintaining Chemical Balance

There are thousands of biochemical reactions going on in the body all of the time. Vitamins and minerals make these reactions possible. Nerve impulses that make feeling and movement possible, enzyme production that makes digestion possible, hormone production, waste removal and even muscle movement are made possible by thousands of chemical reactions that are dependent on balanced biochemistry made possible by proper nutrition. Chemical balance, which makes it possible for the cells of the body to have energy, make their products, eliminate waste and reproduce—is dependent on good nutrition.

It is not as if these reactions completely shut down with an improper diet. If that were true, there would not be an overpopulation problem. We have the capacity to store most nutrients. Our bodies also have a way of prioritizing the use of nutrients. The brain, heart and kidneys are kept running at the expense of other bodily functions when nutrients are in short supply.

A body in a poor nutritional state does not necessarily become diseased in the sense that traditional Western doctors, trained to find pathology, would notice. Pathology usually doesn't develop until many years of neglect. Neglecting health leads to a variety of subclinical complaints such as fatigue, joint pain, frequent colds, allergies, sinusitis, rashes, hives, dry skin, depression, headaches and other health problems.

We are now in the third generation of junk food. Fast food and empty calories have been a way of life since the 1950s. Pollution is getting worse and our soil is becoming depleted of trace nutrients.

Nutritionally depleted parents are having children that are even more nutritionally depleted. As time goes on, nutritional reserves are less for each succeeding generation. Some vague, chronic complaints are now becoming named disease entities, such as chronic fatigue syndrome, fibromyalgia, attention deficit disorder, and hyperactivity in children. It may seem to you that there are more chronically ill children. There are children who have had several courses of antibiotics before the age of five, are obese, have trouble paying attention in school and have behavioral problems. Poor health seems to be increasing.

**Research Can be Flawed**

The symptoms of vitamin deficiency are many and varied. Unfortunately, many doctors are well versed in pharmacology, pathology and surgery, but know less about normal physiology than George W. Bush knows about diction.

You may have seen studies that show glucosamine sulfate and chondroitan sulfate help relieve arthritis symptoms. Although promising, relief from glucosamine or chondroitan sulfate is not seen in 100% of people who take the supplements. One study showed that glucosamine sulfate improved symptoms in 52% of the patients in the study. What about the other 48%? Instead of trying to find one thing to treat the arthritis, it would be better to combine some therapies and try to increase the number of people who favorably respond. In general, patients taking glucosamine or chondroitan products improve, but not 100% of the patients, and the amount of improvement varies from patient to patient. As a general rule, glucosamine or chondroitan products are not as effective as anti-inflammatory drugs—at least initially. As time passes, the glucosamine and chondroitin products surpass the drugs in efficacy. One possible reason is that the drugs contribute to the degeneration of cartilage.

Patients taking glucosamine or chondroitin sulfate would do better if they consumed adequate water, the proper essential fatty acids, avoided processed foods and hydrogenated oils, exercised and were given digestive support where needed. Designing a study where the subjects did everything possible to improve their symptoms would yield interesting results.

Unfortunately, it is unlikely that such a study will be performed because medical studies tend to focus only on single issues. This is why we get such bizarre and conflicting nutritional information from the scientific community. Real scientists, like biophysicists, biochemists and others doing research on living systems, do their research very differently than those doing medical research. Of course these scientists don't sell ads to drug companies in their journals.

Fortunately, health care professionals trained in nutrition understand this and design programs that take into account each and every individual patient. The idea is not to treat arthritis (sinusitis, allergies, digestive problems, reflux, depression, fatigue or any other condition), but rather the patients who have these conditions.

We are not petri dishes. Human beings are so complex. Our biochemistry involves so many variables that tests involving a single aspect of nutrition often do not yield good results. Also, the design and interpretation of scientific studies can lead to conflicting conclusions. It's like the story of the Harvard researcher who was working with frogs. He'd yell and slam a rolled newspaper near the frog. The startled frog would jump. The researcher made the frog jump several times. He took notes, plotted his results on a graph and averaged them out. He found that, on average, the frog jumped 20 feet.

He then cut a leg off of the frog and repeated the experiment. He yelled and slammed the rolled newspaper behind the animal. On average the frog jumped 15 feet.

The researcher repeated the experiment after cutting off another of the frog's legs. On average the frog could jump only 10 feet.

He cut off a third leg, made a very loud noise by yelling and slamming the newspaper. The poor frog struggled, but did manage to jump 5 feet.

After cutting off the last of the frog's legs off, the researcher tried to get it to jump. He yelled louder and louder. He slammed the paper harder and harder, but the frog just lay there. The researcher came to the conclusion that removing all of the legs made the animal hard of hearing.

The point is that research only offers a narrow range of information, which is open to interpretation. There really isn't much difference between studies linking cholesterol consumption with cholesterol levels, and the research involving the frog.

Many may be indignant that the researcher caused the frog so much suffering in the name of science. I felt the same way and tried to contact him, but was unsuccessful. He was pummeled to death with organic carrots by a vegetarian street gang, *The Soys in the 'Hood*.

The double-blind, placebo-controlled model used by medical researchers is being abandoned by other scientists doing research on living systems. Scientists are beginning to understand that there are just too many variables to isolate one thing and expect any kind of coherent result. When research is properly designed to study living systems, the so-called "alternative" therapies begin to look better.

Drugs are much more widely researched than vitamins. One of the reasons is that drugs can be patented, vitamins cannot. The huge profits pharmaceutical companies realize from drug sales are just not possible with vitamins. Drugs can cause massive changes in physiology that more natural substances are incapable of causing, making research on drugs more cut and dried. (Come to think of it, there are natural substances that cause massive changes in physiology, but they're illegal.)

There is a research-driven mythology in this country. The television news likes to use little health tidbits released by researchers. Unfortunately they don't tell you any of the details of the study performed, only the conclusion. For instance, recently a study was performed on children and whether or not sugar was involved with hyperactivity. The children in the experiment were put on additive-free diets and given a measured dose of sugar. Actually, in the study, the researchers gave sugar to their control group. Also, the sugar was given in a single dose. The researchers came to the conclusion that sugar did not affect hyperactivity. Of course the argument can be made that having the children on additive-free diets made them less prone to be hyperactive, but that idea was left out of the news report. The news only reported "Sugar has no effect on hyperactive children." They created a myth. If our frog experiment was reported on the television news, we'd hear, "Frogs hear with their legs, film at 11." When different research is done and comes to different conclusions, we'll hear that. This is why we keep getting conflicting information about health. You are told to eat margarine, then you are told don't eat margarine. It's very confusing. You can't make up your mind so you keep waiting for another news report to straighten things out. Unfortunately, the news doesn't exist to inform you. It exists to entertain you enough to keep you watching so the sponsors can sell you hemorrhoid cream and diet cola.

Another problem is the amount of influence that the drug companies have on which research gets published. They do, after all, buy advertisements in the medical journals. If the journals choose to publish something disparaging about a drug therapy, the company can cause financial harm to the journal by pulling its ads. This is a very strong reason why there is not enough research published to support nutritional therapies. In fact, some research on natural therapies is designed to fail. If I make $3 billion each year selling a drug for ADD, I may not be pleased with your journal if you publish an article that supports giving B vitamin supplementation and avoiding sugar as a way to improve children with ADD, and I can hurt your journal economically by pulling my ads.

The type of research being done in this country, the philosophy of our doctors and a general laziness on our part, are why we have sickness care instead of health care. We fight cancer, heart disease and other diseases, but we don't promote health. It's true that there are new attempts to get Americans to change their lifestyles. These attempts are feeble compared to the efforts that go into developing new drugs and technology to battle disease.

**The Real Problem**

The biggest health problem in America is not cancer or heart disease. We are not lacking in new drugs or technology. The biggest health problem is the fact that so many Americans are tired all of the time. One of the major causes of the fatigue epidemic in this country is poor nutrition. If you solve the problem of fatigue early in life, you will reduce the chances of serious disease later in life.

Inadequate intake of vitamins and minerals can exist for several reasons. Eating a nutrient-deficient, refined diet, alcoholism or drug abuse, poor digestion or absorption, chemical pollution from pesticides and food additives, and even genetic defects can all lead to poor nutritional status.

It is preferable to get your vitamins from nutritious food than to get them from pills. However, deficiencies may make it necessary to take supplements. There are clues that tell you whether you need a particular vitamin.

For instance, if you have been spending years eating a lot of sugar, white flour and not eating whole grains, you probably need vitamin B complex, vitamin C and minerals. People who need vitamin B complex may be fatigued, have low blood pressure, frequently get headaches that feel like a band around their head, and they may fall asleep but have problems staying asleep at night.

If you lack vitamin $B_6$, you won't remember your dreams. If you take $B_6$ and it doesn't help, you may need to take the active form, pyridoxyl-5-phosphate. If you only get help from the active form of $B_6$, it probably means that you need magnesium. When you are outside with a group of people and it seems like you are the only one being bitten by insects, you probably need niacin and riboflavin (vitamin $B_3$ and vitamin $B_2$). People needing folic acid often confuse right and left or transpose letters and numbers when writing. Folic acid is a common deficiency because cooking destroys it.

One good way to tell if you need zinc is to taste zinc sulfate liquid. This is available in a product called *Aqueous Zinc,* which is made by Biotics Research. Taste a capful of the liquid. If you are extremely deficient in zinc, the liquid will be tasteless. If you have a slight deficiency, it will have a slight bitter taste. If you do not need zinc, the liquid will taste bitter and strong. Other signs of zinc deficiency are white spots on the fingernails and patches of dry skin.

People with nails that are brittle and crack frequently need trace minerals. These people may also benefit from a supplement that includes all eight essential amino acids. These deficiencies are often the result of an underproduction of hydrochloric acid in the stomach, known as hypochlorhydra.

Excessive body odor or sweaty feet is often an indication of a need for magnesium. (If your feet smell and your nose runs, you're built upside down.) Also, taking magnesium and $B_6$ can reduce the tendency to get kidney stones.

If you have dry skin, muscle fatigue and dandruff or if you crave greasy foods, you probably need essential fatty acids. Also, if you take aspirin frequently, and it is a good pain reliever for you, essential fatty acid supplementation may help you to get by with less aspirin.

## FOOD

Everything the body does is a chemical reaction, and food is the raw material for these reactions. Your body burns carbohydrate as fuel. Fat is stored, and is used as fuel in times when food is scarce. Fat is also important to the endocrine and the immune system. Protein is used as structural material and to give osmotic pressure to the blood. Adequate protein intake is necessary to remove toxins from the body. Protein is also used as a raw material for enzymes, which are proteins that cause chemical reactions without being changed by the reaction; they are organic catalysts. Protein aids in immunity in the blood and helps the nervous system to work. Vitamins and minerals in your diet act as cofactors to enzymes—sort of like the ignition key in an automobile. They enable the enzymes to function.

Carbohydrates come in two forms—sugar and complex carbohydrates. Sugar is a small molecule. Simple sugars have six carbon molecules. Think of a sugar molecule as a boxcar. A disaccharide is two linked boxcars. Starch, or complex carbohydrate, is like a train, with dozens of boxcars linked together.

Similarly, protein is a long molecule, like a freight train. The smaller molecules making up the boxcars of the protein train are called amino acids. Eight of the 22 amino acids are essential, which means that they cannot be produced by the body and must be eaten in the diet.

Fats are put together a little differently than carbohydrates and proteins. The base molecule for fat is the triglyceride. It is a three-pronged molecule, with glycerol as a base. Attached to each of the prongs of the molecule is a long molecule called a fatty acid.

Sterols are another form of fat that have an entirely different structure than triglycerides. Sterols are ringed molecules. The best known of these is cholesterol. Sterols are important in the formation of hormones.

Digestion is the process of taking each of these large fat, protein and carbohydrate molecules, breaking them down into small molecules and transporting them into the blood stream. Protein is broken down into amino acids. Complex carbohydrates are broken down into sugars. Fat is broken down into fatty acids and glycerin. The small molecules can then be absorbed by the body and used by the cells as raw material.

**Sugar**

Eating refined sugar damages your health and energy. Many people increase their energy simply by giving up refined sugar. Too much sugar is harmful to digestion and nutrient absorption. In your intestines, there is a delicate balance of nature between bacteria and yeast. If you eat a lot of sugar, you create an environment that favors yeast growth. Too much yeast can cause a lot of problems. You may tend to bloat or get tired when you eat. You may develop allergies. Many women become prone to vaginal yeast infections. Ironically, yeast overgrowth can make you crave sugar.

Eating refined sugar is also hard on the endocrine system. It puts stress on the pancreas and on the adrenal glands, causing fatigue. If you are tired and you eat a lot of sugar, give it up and you'll feel better.

Refined sugar is addictive. Eating it causes a sudden increase in your blood sugar, which scares the heck out of your pancreas. Your pancreas hasn't evolved since Neolithic times and hasn't the foggiest idea of what a Twix bar is. You have the pancreas of a caveman, and it responds to the increase in your blood sugar as if you'd just eaten a bushel of potatoes. It makes enough insulin to respond to a future need. Unfortunately, the increase in blood sugar from the Twix bar you just ate is short-lived. You end up with extra insulin circulating through your bloodstream. Your body interprets this as wanting more sugar. The cravings are pretty strong, and many people have trouble giving up sugar.

Excess insulin is created by overconsumption of sugar and causes health problems. For one thing, insulin moves fat into the cells; so if you want to get fat, eat sugar and produce a lot of insulin. One of the reasons the low-fat diet craze was such a miserable failure was because people began eating huge amounts of starch (white bread, noodles etc.), which your body treats exactly the same way that it treats sugar. Eating starch increases insulin and causes the body to store fat.

Over time, if you keep eating refined foods, your body becomes insensitive to insulin. This situation, if left unchecked, leads to type II diabetes. The body produces plenty of insulin, but it doesn't respond to the insulin and the blood sugar goes up.

Another long-term problem caused by excess consumption of sugar and starch is high cholesterol and high triglycerides. This is the so-called "Syndrome X." In Syndrome X, the cholesterol is high, the LDL (bad cholesterol) is high, the HDL (good cholesterol) is low and the triglycerides are high. The patient is usually overweight and may have insulin insensitivity and high blood pressure. These patients will go on low-fat diets that will have very little effect on their cholesterol levels. Many times they are placed on a drug to lower their cholesterol. One of the ways that some of these cholesterol-lowering drugs work is to suppress an enzyme in the liver called HMGCoA reductase. HMGCoA reductase is stimulated by insulin. Sugar consumption helps to increase cholesterol.

Your health care provider trained in nutrition can help you to read your blood test and know if this situation exists. This Syndrome X pattern can be seen in so called "normal" blood tests by someone who knows what to look for.

Treating Syndrome X or type II diabetes should include eating a low-glycemic diet. A low-glycemic diet is one where the foods consumed do not trigger much insulin production. One such diet that rose to recent popularity is *Sugar Busters*. Supplementation with a multivitamin designed to lower blood sugar is also very helpful. One such product is GlucoBalance, which is made by Biotics Research. Other supple-mentation may also be helpful. You may need adrenal support, essential fatty acids, liver support or other nutrients to make your program more effective. You should see a health professional trained in nutritional therapy and have your individual needs addressed.

Bringing sugar cravings under control is easier than most people realize. Many can usually bring their cravings under control within a day or two. You absolutely do not want to skip meals—especially breakfast. The key is not to go more than two hours without snacking. If lunch is at noon and dinner at six, eat something at two and at four. Protein is your best choice; raw nuts are particularly good. Fruit is acceptable as a snack, sugary or starchy snacks are not.

Chewing your food thoroughly also will help to control sugar cravings. Chewing improves digestion and absorption of nutrients, bringing hunger and food cravings under control.

Sugar is addictive, and sometimes changing your eating patterns does not ensure that the cravings will go away. Once again, supplementation can help here. Biotics Research makes a multivitamin designed for people who become hypoglycemic and crave sugar. It is called Bio-Glycozyme Forte.

Problems with digestion and absorption may make it difficult to give up sugar. Refined sugar is very easily absorbed. It is much easier to digest and absorb than protein or even whole grains. Even people with digestion and absorption problems absorb sugar easily. People who do not digest protein or other nutrients very well, crave sugar. Unconsciously, they understand that they will get *some* nutrient out of that Hershey bar. They may even be aware that they don't feel very well when they eat wholesome foods. You see this a lot in older people. They don't care much for meat, but they love desserts.

As people get older, they produce less hydrochloric acid for digestion, making it more difficult to digest protein. Some believe this is why people get osteoarthritis. The body needs protein to sustain life. The brain, kidneys, heart and other vital organs all need protein. When there is a lack of protein (in this case because of a problem digesting protein), the body has a priority system deciding where the protein goes. It will steal the protein from less important areas, such as joint surfaces, for use in areas that are vital for survival.

Joint movement is not as important as kidney, heart or brain function. (Well, maybe joint movement is more important than brain function in Congressmen, career government bureaucrats and certain NFL draft picks.) In order to survive, the body sacrifices ease of movement, which is a luxury compared to these other functions.

Allergies can also make it difficult to give up sugar. Often someone who can't give up sugar has an allergy to corn (and therefore corn syrup, one of the more common sweeteners), cane sugar or even chocolate. People who are allergic to a food tend to be addicted to it, much the same way an alcoholic is addicted. In fact Dr. Theron Randolph (noted allergist and a man who can be considered the founder of clinical ecology), called alcoholism the ultimate food allergy.

Eating refined sugar makes the adrenal glands overwork in order to keep the blood sugar level. Refined sugar overworks the pancreas, and causes major problems with digestion and with the general health of the digestive tract. Refined sugar creates nutrient deficiencies and causes fatigue in so many different ways that you cannot reasonably expect to feel energetic unless you eliminate refined sugar from your diet.

**The Importance of Whole Grains**

Because of Americans' paranoia about fat, pasta was, for a long time, lauded as a health food. Pasta is low in fat, but most pasta is made with refined white flour. Filling up on white bread and noodles because they are low in fat is a lot like eating road apples because they don't have cyanide. Two-by-fours are low in fat, but you wouldn't want to eat one with a mess of marinara sauce, would you? Just because one aspect of dietary advice is good, doesn't make everything about it good. The Atkins diet correctly gets people to stop eating refined carbohydrates, but doesn't have a problem with recommending all kinds of unhealthy fats. The argument put forth by fans of the Atkins diet is that it is better to eat that way than to eat all of the carbohydrates that Americans consume. It is better to break your leg than to stab yourself in the eye. That doesn't make breaking your leg a good thing.

Eating refined white flour products causes some of the same problems that eating sugar causes. Refined white flour is broken down and absorbed very quickly, much like sugar. It also causes the same changes in bowel pH as sugar does. This creates an imbalance in bowel flora, killing normal flora and allowing pathogenic flora to exist. Normal bowel flora detoxifies xenobiotics, manufactures vitamins, and helps keep the intestinal lining healthy.

In nature, anything that contains complex carbohydrates also contains some vitamin B, vitamin E and fiber. Interestingly, B vitamins aid in carbohydrate metabolism. When you eat whole grains, you are automatically consuming the vitamins you need to process them.

Some refined products are labeled *enriched,* which is a great piece of doublespeak that would make George Orwell proud. Enriching means that the manufacturer takes all of the B vitamins, vitamin E, essential fatty acids and fiber out of the grain, then puts back some of the B vitamins. Let me borrow $100. I'll give you $5 back and tell you that I enriched your money.

Let's say that someone stole your BMW (Oops, the '80s are over, I mean your Lexus. Oops, the '90s are over, I mean your SUV.) The police find it. The thieves have stripped the car completely; they've taken the stereo, the cellular phone, the leather seats, the quarter panels, the tires and the engine. They even took your tollbooth change and your Barry Manilow CD. The thieves decided that they wanted to drive the frame. They put in mismatched tires, a bucket seat from an old AMC Pacer, a gas tank from a 1973 Pinto and an engine from an old Desoto. The door is being held closed with a bungi cord and your Barry Manilow CD is being used for an ashtray. The police call you and tell you that they've located your *enriched* automobile. That loaf of white bread has been *enriched* in a similar manner.

Eat foods the way nature created them. There is a good deal of misinformation circulating about nutrition. People tend to think in terms of RDAs and absolute amounts of nutrients. Most of the vitamins were discovered in the 1930s when chemical know-how wasn't very sophisticated. For example, as far as the government is concerned, ascorbic acid is vitamin C; but a food that is high in vitamin C has much more in it than just ascorbic acid. Food containing vitamin C complex has bioflavonoids, vitamin K and other nutrients. Eating food that is high in vitamin C is different from taking ascorbic acid.

Vitamin B complex is present in foods that contain complex carbohydrates. The B vitamins in these foods exist in very definite proportions to each other and to certain synergistic minerals that enable them to be absorbed by your body. These important combinations are never taken into consideration when manufacturers *enrich* their products.

The chemistry of the living cell and the human body is much more complex than the chemistry that takes place in a lab or a beaker. Biomolecules work like little factories or fine machinery. You can give a chemist a Rolex watch, and he or she can analyze it and tell you how much gold, glass, quartz and other materials are in it. You can take the same watch and smash it with a hammer and, from the chemist's point of view, nothing has changed. Cellulose and starch have the same chemical formula. Chemically, there is no difference between wood and a potato, except how the molecule is arranged. Many things added to foods, put there by manufacturers as nutrients, are as useful to the body as wood.

Complex carbohydrates in nature always contain fiber. Fiber is cellulose from the cell walls of plants. You cannot digest and absorb it. Other nutrients adhere to fiber and are absorbed more slowly than they would be if there was no fiber in the meal. It sort of makes your meal time-released. The gradual absorption of whole grain is not nearly as much of a burden on your pancreas as the rapid absorption of refined grains. White bread and pasta are rapidly absorbed, causing the blood sugar to increase, stressing the pancreas.

The fiber in whole grains also cuts down on the number of calories and fat you absorb from your food. It makes your bowel healthy and reduces your chances of getting cancer by increasing bowel motility and reducing the toxicity of the bowel. Normal bowel bacteria feed on fiber, so a diet that is high in fiber helps keep the bowel healthy. White bread has no fiber.

You own the body of a prehistoric hunter-gatherer. Food technology has changed faster than your body's ability to adapt to those changes. Your body has not adapted to eating starch or sugar that is not consumed with vitamins and fiber. Sugars or complex carbohydrates eaten in their natural state, with the fiber, are absorbed slowly. White flour and sugar are absorbed more quickly than anything your prehistoric ancestors had.

Eating refined foods makes the pancreas produce insulin at a very rapid rate. The pancreas overproduces insulin and causes a hypoglycemic state. You end up with all of that extra insulin and nothing for it to do except lower the blood sugar, making your crave more sweets or starch.

These blood sugar swings are hard on your endocrine system. They are stressful. Physiologically, your body doesn't know the difference between this stress and having Attila the Hun for a boss, a cheating spouse or a certified letter from Adolph Q. Sphincter of the IRS suggesting you show up at their offices with your 1994–2001 income tax records. The stress of blood sugar swings is one reason why refined foods cause fatigue.

The stress of eating incorrectly is as tiring as the stress of worrying, physically exhausting yourself or not sleeping. Your endocrine system simply doesn't know the difference.

People in primitive societies, who are suddenly exposed to modern diets, experience a dramatic increase in health problems. Jonathan Wright, MD, in his book *Dr. Wright's Guide to Healing with Nutrition*, has several examples of the deterioration of the health of primitive people after adopting a modern diet. The most notable change in their diet was an increase in sugar and other refined carbohydrates. One example in Dr. Wright's book is the Eskimos living in Northern Canada. It is taken from an article by Otto Schaefer, entitled "When the Eskimo Comes to Town," which appeared in the November/December 1971 issue of *Nutrition Today*. The Eskimos studied had no exposure to civilization until the 1940s. Within 10 years of the dietary change, the number of diabetics tripled. Five times as many men over 40 developed diseases of the arteries. Gallbladder surgery, which was never necessary for these people, became common. Teenagers developed acne, and some women developed breast cancer, maladies which were unheard of prior to 1940.

Sugar and other refined carbohydrates undermine your health and energy level, much the same way that it destroyed the health of the Canadian Eskimos. The only difference is we have had this diet for so long that we aren't aware of the damage it is causing.

## Fresh Fruits and Vegetables

You should have a minimum of four cups of fresh vegetables and three pieces of fruit every day. Have more, if you like. Fruit and vegetables are high in bulk and fiber and will improve your digestion, speed up your bowel transit time, nourish your normal bowel flora and decrease the toxicity in your colon. Your health and energy will increase and your chances for developing bowel cancer will decrease.

If you are constipated, there is a very good chance that your lack of energy is linked to your bowel. It is very important that you eat enough fresh produce. Drinking plenty of water and eating plenty of fruits and vegetables will cure most cases of constipation.

Digesting food takes a lot of energy. Those people with inefficient digestive systems use more energy than those who digest well. The bulk, fiber and enzymatic help from fresh fruits and vegetables will improve your digestion and eliminate a major source of fatigue.

Fruits and vegetables are also rich in vitamins and minerals and low in calories. Nutritional deficiency is a major cause of fatigue. Those who don't eat fresh produce often suffer from fatigue due to a lack of certain nutrients. Eating fresh fruits and vegetables provides plenty of nutrients, makes the body's chemistry function optimally and increases energy.

## Raw Foods

Americans eat too much cooked food. Food that is cooked requires all of the digestive enzymes to be produced by the body. Cooked food is harder to digest than raw food. Raw fruits and vegetables contain enzymes that aid digestion. There are those who believe that we live off of the energy from the food we eat and not the chemical constituents of it and that nothing but live, raw food is good.

Cooking also destroys some vitamins. Heat destroys thiamin ($B_1$), riboflavin ($B_2$), folic acid, vitamin C and pantothenic acid ($B_5$). Pantothenic acid is destroyed by heat in the presence of an acid or alkali. It is stable in neutral solutions.

Vitamins $B_5$ and $B_6$ can be destroyed by light. Vitamin $B_{12}$ and folic acid are easily oxidized to a form not usable by the body. Other vitamins can be destroyed by either alkaline or acid pH. Even exposure to light can destroy certain nutrients.

This is not to say that you should avoid cooked food. You should just try to eat some raw vegetables or fruit with every meal. Food is always best in its natural state.

## ADDITIVES, AGRIBUSINESS AND THE OTHER SIDE OF POOR NUTRITION

Even if you are eating what you think is a good diet, you may not be getting enough of certain vitamins, and you may be consuming a lot of toxic substances. Your diet can be causing fatigue and other health problems without your being aware of it. The average American consumes 10 pounds of food additives per year. This is just additives that the food industry purposely puts in food. This doesn't count the insecticides, fungicides, herbicides and other chemicals used by farmers.

Processing, even simple cooking, decreases the nutritional value of food. Boiling leaches vitamins and minerals out of the food and into the cooking water. Certain vitamins are not stable to heat.

Food manufacturers and processors do not pay attention to the nutritional content of the foods they prepare. They are more concerned with taste, shelf life, texture and appearance. Processed food is a victory of form over substance.

A variety of chemicals are added to food to preserve it and to give it desirable texture, firmness and consistency. Sugar and fat are added to enhance the food's desirability and to mask the taste of the additives. There is even a chemical to help hide the taste of the other chemicals. The manufacturers want the consumer to perceive their products as real food that has the qualities we value in food, even if it is chemically laden and valueless. A little bit of chemical know-how and voila! You have a "food" that can stay on your grocer's shelf until the Second Coming, and still be edible. (Well, sellable anyway; it probably never was edible.)

Thousands of years from now, archaeologists will find a package of Mostess Winkies in some ruins. The cakes will still be soft and edible (or at least not any less edible than they were when they were manufactured). Scientists will marvel at this discovery. Much will be said about our culture's ability to embalm food. Some of the scientists will postulate that the food was meant to be buried with kings to supply them with nutrients on their long trip to the underworld. The Winkies will be sold at auction for a small fortune, like wine found in ancient Roman ruins is sold today.

Many patients, after being advised about how harmful additives are, ask if frozen dinners are healthy. They see the labels on frozen foods and find them to be relatively chemical-free—for convenience foods. The problem is that if these are eaten frequently, the diet becomes very deficient in vitamin C and most of the B vitamins.

Researchers at Rutgers University measured the levels of vitamin C in a frozen chicken pot pie. They couldn't find any. They then added a known amount of vitamin C to the thawed pie, refroze it and heated it. Two days later they found that this process destroyed about 25% of the vitamin C.

Frozen foods, while having fewer chemicals than many other processed foods, tend to be vitamin deficient. There are nutrients, like minerals, that are stable, and not affected by freezing and reheating. Frozen food is sometimes an acceptable compromise for someone who is busy. It is not a good idea to have frozen dinners every day. Frozen food is, however, better for you than many of the additive-laden foods people eat every day. If you eat a lot of frozen dinners, supplement with a good multiple vitamin (Bio-Multi Plus from Biotics is a good product) and try to snack on raw vegetables. Raw foods contain enzymes and folic acid. Many health experts believe that we do not get enough "live" food (like fresh, raw produce) and that live food provides health benefits that go beyond providing necessary vitamins and minerals.

Compare the bread that is sold to the American public to the bread that was consumed by primitive societies. It will give you an idea of how technology has undermined health. The ancient Egyptians developed the technique of grinding grain between two stones. The technique produced flour that could be made into cohesive dough. Since that time, light-colored bread has been prized. The more bran that is removed, the whiter the bread. The light-colored bread of ancient times still had some of the bran and all of the wheat germ. Ancient societies did not have the technology to completely strip the nutrients from grain. We have that technology today. Modern white flour is completely striped of nutrients. It has none of the germ, which contains vitamin E and octocosinol. It has none of the bran, which contains the B vitamins and fiber.

Modern bakers were inconvenienced by the fact that the baking qualities of flour varied from batch to batch. Consistency between batches has been achieved by bleaching the flour with chlorine gas.

Bleached flour is a much more workable product for the mechanized food industry.

43

Unfortunately, chlorine does more than bleach and mature the flour. It interacts with the other molecules in the flour, creating things like the chlorinated lipid and dichlorostearic acid. Another bleaching agent, nitrogen trichloride, reacts with methionine residues and forms methionine sulfoximine, which can cause nervous seizures, similar to epilepsy. The chlorine also destroys any vitamin E that may be left in the flour.

Modern commercial bread frequently has added mono and diglycerides in order to make it soft. If you add a little potassium bromate, you can whip up the bread and cause it to rise in as little as two minutes. Never mind the fact that potassium bromate is a deadly poison; it's a small price to pay for increased production, efficiency and consistency between batches. Of course now our modern product has five chemicals added and all of the nutrients removed—and you're wondering why you're tired.

Here is the list of ingredients of a typical loaf of modern white bread: enriched all purpose flour, enzyme active soy preparation, salt, sugar, lard, skim milk powder, monoglycerides, diglycerides, calcium proprionate, yeast food (containing flour, salt calcium sulfate, ammonium chloride and potassium bromate), benzoyl peroxide, niacin, iron, tricalcium phosphate, potassium bromate, thiamine mononitrite, and magnesium carbonate.

In exchange for the fiber, vitamin E, octocosinol and vitamin B complex removed from the bread, the manufacturer has added a half dozen chemicals and two B vitamins. The *experts* in charge of telling the American public about nutrition, after much debate, have decided to tell us to eat according to a *food pyramid* and to get plenty of grains. Unfortunately, they make no distinction between the garbage listed above and whole grains.

Look in Ruth Winters' *Consumer's Dictionary of Food Additives,* to learn what some of the stuff that's been added to the bread is.

*Mono and diglycerides:* Used to maintain softness. Diglycerides are on the FDA list of food additives to be studied for possible mutagenic, teratogenic, subacute and reproductive effects. This is medicalese for birth defects, cancer and reproductive problems.

*Calcium proprionate:* Mold inhibitor, generally regarded as safe by the FDA.

*Benzoyl peroxide:* A bleaching agent; also skin irritant and possible allergen. Benzoyl peroxide is toxic if inhaled. Generally regarded as safe by the FDA. It's used in acne cream.

*Tricalcium phosphate:* An anticaking agent and a dietary supplement with no known toxicity.

*Potassium bromate:* Used to obtain a fine, spongelike quality in the bread. Legal allowance is 50 ppb (ppb = parts per billion). Very toxic when taken internally. Between two and four ounces of a 2% bromine solution can poison a child. Burns and skin irritation have been reported from its industrial uses. In 1980 the Ames test found potassium bromate to be a mutagen. Dr. Bruce Ames, a biochemist at the University of California in the early 1970s, developed the Ames test. He used bacteria that reveal whether a chemical is a mutagen, one that causes genetic changes in the bacteria. Almost all chemicals that are known carcinogens have also shown to be mutagenic on the Ames test. Whether the test can identify carcinogens is still controversial (much the same way the "Flat Earth Society" finds the idea that the world is round, controversial, or that the tobacco industry finds the link between smoking and lung cancer, controversial).

*Magnesium carbonate:* Generally regarded as safe.

*Calcium sulfate:* Plaster of Paris. (Helluva thing to find in bread, isn't it?) Calcium sulfate is used as a firming agent, yeast food and dough conditioner. Because it absorbs moisture and hardens quickly, its ingestion may result in intestinal obstruction. Mixed with flour, it has been used to kill rodents. Generally regarded as safe by the FDA.

*Ammonium chloride:* Dough conditioner and yeast food. Naturally occurring and generally regarded as safe by the FDA.

In a 110-pound batch of bread there is about 75 grams of additives, not counting the vitamins added to *enrich* the product. It's about three ounces of chemical, a little less than one gram per loaf. Some are harmful; some are not so harmful, according to the FDA. You many think that this is not a lot to consume; the FDA certainly doesn't. Unfortunately, the studies that allow the chemicals to be placed in food are done on animals, one chemical at a time. There are no studies on the cumulative effects of all of the additives. Also, this amount is not including the chemicals produced when the natural ingredients of the bread interact with the additives, such as dichlorostearic acid and methionine sulfoximine.

Let's say that you have this bread for lunch. You have a bologna sandwich, made with low-fat turkey bologna, because you're health conscious. You have a diet orange soda because you want to avoid sugar and caffeine, and you're watching your weight. You have a salad made of iceberg lettuce because the American Cancer Society finally got around to recommending fruits and vegetables after spending decades telling you that diet has nothing to do with cancer.

Your diet orange soda has aspartame (Nutrasweet), citric acid, sodium benzoate, gum acacia, natural flavors, glycerol, ester of wood rosin, yellow #6, brominated vegetable oil, and red #40. Winter's book, *A Consumer's Dictionary of Food Additives* is an excellent resource for finding out what exactly the chemicals are in your food. Information about additives have been obtained form other sources as well, including David Steinman's book, *Diet for a Poisoned Planet,* and Kirk Hamilton's publication *Clinical Pearls*. Let's take a look at some of these ingredients.

*Aspartame:* Sold under the brand names Nutrasweet and Equal. This was approved by the FDA for limited use, in crystalline form in 1981. Approval came over the objections of a federal panel that wanted further testing to examine a possible link between brain cancer and aspartame. Indeed, there has been an increase in brain cancer since aspartame's approval. Some experts believe there may be a link between aspartame and headaches, anxiety attacks, memory loss, breathing difficulty, heart palpitations, nausea, seizures and blurred vision. Aspartame also raises the pH of urine, creating a tendency for the user to get bladder infections.

There have been some studies that seem to indicate that there is no connection between seizures and aspartame use; however, these have utilized the crystalline form of aspartame, given in a single dosage. Aspartame, when heated or in liquid, releases methanol, which is poisonous. Also, aspartame users take it in small doses throughout the day. There needs to be more studies, but these researchers have currently occupied themselves with studying hearing in frogs.

*Sodium benzoate:* A preservative that has been around for a long time. No known toxicity.

*Gum acacia:* Used to retard sugar crystallization. Also used as a foam stabilizer in soft drinks. Generally regarded as safe by the FDA. Gum acacia causes allergic reactions in some people.

*Natural flavors:* According to Ruth Winter's book, the FDA considers something natural if it involves only minimal processing, such as peeling, homogenizing, baking and other things that can be done in the kitchen. Also the food cannot have anything synthetic or any added chemicals. Beyond that, you don't know what these natural flavors are.

*Ester of wood rosin:* Wood rosin is the exudate from a living southern pine tree; it has no known toxicity. Ester is a compound formed from the rosin to reduce its allergy-causing properties.

*Yellow #6:* Possible link to kidney and adrenal tumors. Yellow #6 has been banned in Norway and Sweden.

*Brominated vegetable oil:* Used as an emulsifier. The FDA has it on the suspect list. Bromates are highly toxic. They can cause death through kidney failure or nervous system problems. Bromates can inhibit the body's defenses. Between two and four ounces of a 2% solution can poison a child. Also, severe allergic reactions have been reported. Brominated vegetable oil has also been found in human fat tissue, which means that the body stores this poison.

*Red #40:* Suspected carcinogen. Whenever you see a color followed by a number, avoid that food.

Your low-fat bologna has added: dextrose, hydrogenated milk protein, sodium phosphate, sodium erythrobate and sodium nitrite.

*Dextrose:* Corn sugar.

***Hydrogenated milk protein:*** Generally regarded as safe by the FDA.

***Sodium phosphate:*** Generally regarded as safe by the FDA.

***Sodium erythrobate:*** An antioxidant with no known toxicity.

***Sodium nitrite:*** Makes meat bright red and kills Clostridium Botulinum spores (botulism). Nitrite combines with natural stomach chemicals and chemicals in the food to form nitrosamines, which are *powerful carcinogens.*

Isn't it interesting that nitrites are known carcinogens? That's right, ***known carcinogens,*** not suspected, not just some suspicious tests. We know that nitrates create a chemical in the stomach that causes cancer. There isn't even a warning label on these products. The FDA has taken the view that nitrites kill botulism spores and there is nothing to take the place of nitrites. Still, it seems odd that the FDA wouldn't have the manufacturers warn the parents who give their children bologna sandwiches and hot dogs for lunch that they may be giving their children cancer. I'm sure that the processed meat industry, being a $125 billion per year industry, had nothing to do with the FDA's decision. This is the same FDA that banned tryptophan because of one brand that was contaminated.

You use a commercial dressing, a low-fat one, since you're watching your weight. Here are the ingredients of a typical low-fat ranch dressing: Water, partially hydrogenated soybean oil, cultured nonfat buttermilk solids, sugar, modified food starch, salt, natural flavors, sodium caseinate; vinegar, phosphoric acid, onion (dehydrated), garlic (dehydrated), monosodium glutamate (enhances flavor [actually tricks your nervous system into thinking that it tastes good]), propylene glycol alginate, mono and diglycerides, sorbic acid, lactic acid, spice, artificial flavor, xanthan gum, disodium inositate and disodium guanylate, parsley (dehydrated), calcium disodium EDTA, THBQ and citric acid.

Here's a synopsis of the ingredients:

*Water:* The most plentiful ingredient in this product. This is a product that advertises itself to be 91% fat free. Since the manufacturer is talking about volume and not total calories, this can be accomplished by watering down the dressing. What's an easy way to make something that's 20% fat into something that's 10% fat? Double the volume by adding water.

*Partially hydrogenated soybean oil:* Hydrogenation turns an unsaturated fat into a saturated one. It changes the configuration of the fat molecule, creating something known as a trans fatty acid. On a molecular level, this is like turning a right-handed glove into a left-handed one. The result is something that can't really be used by the body. Trans fatty acids are actually worse than useless. They interfere with normal fat metabolism and have been linked to heart disease. They have a half-life in the body of 51 days. This means that it takes 51 days for your body to get rid of half of the trans fatty acids you eat. In other words, after 51 days, half of this hydrogenated oil is still in your system. In another 51 days you'll still have one-fourth of it. After another 51 days (153 days total) you'll still have one-eighth of the trans fatty acids in your system.

*Cultured nonfat buttermilk solids:* Probably better than illiterate nonfat buttermilk solids. Actually, it's much like powdered milk.

*Modified food starch:* This is starch that has been chemically altered to make it water soluble. Several different chemicals are used, such as propylene oxide, succinic anhydride, 1-octenyl succinic anhydride, aluminum sulfate, and sodium hydroxide. You have no way of knowing what was used. In David Steinman's book, *Diet for a Poisoned Planet*, he expresses concern about aluminum sulfate being used to modify food starch because there is a possible link between aluminum and Alzheimer's disease.

*Natural flavors:* Flavor from food that has had only minimal processing, without anything synthetic or any added chemical.

*Sodium caseinate:* This is the principle protein of cow's milk.

*Vinegar:* Finally, something you can recognize as a food that you would find in your own kitchen.

*Phosphoric acid:* This is an acid made from phosphate rock. The FDA considers it safe. Steinman makes the point that you can clean rust off of a chrome bumper with it.

*Salt:* Something else that is familiar. Since the connection between Alzheimer's disease and aluminum has been mentioned, you may want to read the label on your table salt. You'll notice that it contains aluminum (sodium silico aluminate) as an anticaking agent. Sea salt, kosher salt and pickling salt are all free of aluminum.

*Onion and garlic:* Good God! More food, this could get to be a habit.

*Monosodium glutamate:* Also known as MSG, which causes "Chinese restaurant syndrome" (chest pain, numbness and headache after eating). MSG causes brain damage in young rodents. Female animals treated with MSG had fewer pregnancies and smaller litters.

*Propylene glycol alginate:* Derived from seaweed. The FDA considers it safe.

*Mono and diglycerides:* Used as stabilizers and emulsifiers. According to Steinman, these can occur in nature, but are usually synthetically made. In his book, Steinman cites studies that show certain types of mono and diglycerides have caused decreased growth in mice, others have caused enlarged kidneys and decrease in the size of testes. (The poor mice probably were not sure whether they were coming or going.)

*Sorbic acid:* This is acetic acid. It is harmless.

*Lactic acid:* This occurs naturally in sour milk. The FDA regards it as safe.

*Spice:* It now has sugar and spice (and everything nice?).

*Artificial flavor:* By definition, something not found in nature, although it may have components that are found in nature. Whatever it is, the manufacturer has opted not to tell you in detail what the substance is. It's sort of a mystery chemical.

*Xanthan gum:* Produced by fermentation of corn sugar. Xanthan gum thickens and helps the dressing to pour well. No known toxicity.

*Disodium inositate:* A flavor enhancer. No known toxicity.

*Parsley:* Another food.

*Calcium disodium EDTA:* Ethylenediaminetetraacetate. No kidding, the kids didn't just play with the keyboard.

EDTA is used to bind materials that are undesirable in food. It hides metallic tastes and other undesirable flavors and colors in the food. This means that the dressing might taste a little weird without the EDTA (small wonder).

*THBQ:* Tertiarybutylhydroquinone. Food manufacturers had a hard time getting this approved, which means that even the FDA wasn't sure it should be on the market. Think about that. According to Ruth Winter's book, death has occurred from ingestion of five grams (about one-fifth of an ounce). Eating one gram can cause nausea, vomiting, ringing in the ears, delirium, a sense of suffocation and collapse. But hey, now the dressing can have a long shelf life.

*Citric acid:* One of the safer additives.

In a typical lunch of a sandwich and salad, here's a list of the harmful chemicals you consume: Mono and diglycerides (possible mutagens); benzoyl peroxide (irritant, acne medicine); potassium bromate (poison, possible carcinogen); calcium sulfate (plaster of Paris); ammonium chloride (safe, but one gram can cause vomiting and nausea); brominated vegetable oil (deadly poison, stored in the body); yellow #6 (possible link to kidney and adrenal tumors); red #40 (possible carcinogen); sodium nitrite (known carcinogen); partially hydrogenated oil (harms fat metabolism, linked to heart disease); aspartame (linked to brain cancer and other health problems); modified food starch (possibly harmful it aluminum was used, you have no way of knowing); EDTA (to help hide the weird taste of the other chemicals); THBQ (deadly poison), and a host of nonharmful chemicals. *Bon appetite!*

If this is a typical lunch for you, is it any wonder that you're tired? Is there any wonder why the cost of health care has skyrocketed? Are you still surprised that the average American consumes 10 pounds of chemical additives each year? Get yourself a copy of *A Consumer's Dictionary of Food Additives*, and take a walk through your supermarket reading labels. You'll be amazed at what you used to consume.

Let's consider an alternative lunch. We'll still have a sandwich. We'll even use a commercially available bread, whole wheat bread from "Natural Ovens of Manitowoc, Wisconsin". Here's a list of ingredients in a loaf of their 100% whole grain bread: Stone ground whole wheat flour, flax seed, oat bran, wheat germ, barley malt, canola oil, yeast, sea salt and honey. We'll have a salad since we're listening to the American Cancer Society. Our second salad will be made with spinach and the dressing will be plain olive oil (extra virgin) and vinegar. Instead of bologna, we will have turkey breast. Instead of a diet soft drink, we will have water. Our second lunch has no chemical additives.

Even if chemicals were not a consideration in the first lunch, it still would not be as good as our second lunch. Compare the vitamin and mineral content of the two lunches.

## A Tale of Two Sandwiches

### Lunch #1—Bologna on white bread with a lettuce salad

| Nutrient | Bread | Bologna | Lettuce | Total |
|----------|-------|---------|---------|-------|
| Calories | 128 | 214.2 | 15 | 357.2 |
| Fat | 1.8 g | 16.1 g | 0 | 17.9 g |
| Protein | 4.0 g | 14.0 g | 1.0 g | 19.0 g |
| Carbohydrate | 23.0 g | 2.14 g | 2.0 g | 27.14 g |
| Vitamin $B_1$ | 0.11 mg | 0.036 mg | 0.05 mg | 0.196 mg |

**Lunch #1 cont'**

| Nutrient | Bread | Bologna | Lettuce | Total |
|---|---|---|---|---|
| Vitamin B$_2$ | 0.14 mg | 0.18 mg | 0.05 mg | 0.23 mg |
| Folic acid | 0 | 0 | 55 mcg | 55 mcg |
| Niacin | 1.8 mg | 3.9 mg | 0 | 5.7 mg |
| Pantothenic acid | 0.2 mg | 0 | 0.05 mg | 0.25 mg |
| Vitamin B$_6$ | 0 | 0.18 mg | 0.05 mg | 0.23 mg |
| Vitamin B$_{12}$ | 0 | 0.44 mcg | 0 | 0.44 mcg |
| Sodium | 52 mg | 792 mg | 10 mg | 854 mg |
| Potassium | 52 mg | 189 mg | 160 mg | 401 mg |
| Calcium | 60 mg | 92.8 mg | 20 mg | 172.8 mg |
| Magnesium | 10 mg | 14.3 mg | 10 mg | 34.3 mg |
| Zinc | 0.3 mg | 2.3 mg | 0.2 mg | 2.8 mg |
| Phosphorus | 52 mg | 157 mg | 20 mg | 229 mg |
| Iron | 1.36 mg | 1.29 mg | 0.5 mg | 3.15 mg |
| Vitamin A (IU) | 0 | 0 | 330 IU | 330 IU |
| Vitamin E (IU) | 0 | 0 | 0.35 IU | 0.35 IU |
| Essential fatty acids | 0 | 0 | 0 | 0 |
| Vitamin C | 0 | 0 | 5 mg | 5 mg |
| Manganese | 0 | 0 | 0.15 mg | 0.15 mg |

## Lunch #2—Turkey on whole wheat with a spinach salad

| Nutrient | Bread | Turkey | Spinach | Total |
|---|---|---|---|---|
| Calories | 140 | 157 | 24 | 311 |
| Fat | 2 g | 3.2 g | 0 | 5.2 g |
| Protein | 9 g | 29.9 g | 3.2 g | 42.1 g |
| Carbohydrate | 33 g | 0 | 4 g | 37 g |
| Vitamin B$_1$ | 0.35 mg | 0.6 mg | 0.1 mg | 1.05 mg |
| Vitamin B$_2$ | 0.17 mg | 0.13 mg | 0.2 mg | 0.5 mg |
| Folic acid | 80 mcg | 6 mcg | 220 mcg | 306 mcg |
| Niacin | 3.8 mg | 6.8 mg | 1.0 mg | 11.6 mg |
| Pantothenic acid | 0.2 mg | 0.68 mg | 0.1 mg | 0.98 mg |
| Vitamin B$_6$ | 0.88 mg | 0.54 mg | 0.24 mg | 1.66 mg |
| Vitamin B$_{12}$ | 0.45 mcg | 0.37 mcg | 0 | 0.82 mcg |
| Sodium | 100 mg | 63 mg | 108 mg | 271 mg |
| Potassium | 200 mg | 285 mg | 624 mg | 1109 mg |
| Calcium | 160 mg | 21 mg | 112 mg | 293 mg |
| Magnesium | 35 mg | 26 mg | 88 mg | 139 mg |
| Zinc | 3.8 mg | 2 mg | 0.6 mg | 6.4 mg |
| Phosphorus | 160 mg | 208 mg | 56 mg | 424 mg |
| Iron | 0 | 1.4 mg | 3.1 mg | 4.5 mg |
| Vitamin A (IU) | 0 | 0 | 7200 IU | 7200 IU |
| Vitamin E (IU) | 1 IU | 0 | 2.7 IU | 3.7 IU |
| Essential fatty acids | 600 mg | 0 | 600 mg | 600 mg |
| Vitamin C | 0 | 32 mg | 32 mg | 32 mg |
| Manganese | 0.6 mg | 0.02 mg | 1.0 mg | 1.62 mg |

Consider the nutritional differences between these two meals. Meal #2 has more than six times as much vitamin C as meal #1. It has 50% more riboflavin; seven times as much vitamin $B_6$; five times as much $B_1$; over 21 times as much vitamin A; 50% more calcium; about four times as much magnesium; twice as much niacin; almost 10 times as much vitamin E; two and a half times as much zinc; four times as much pantothenic acid; six times as much folic acid; twice as much vitamin $B_{12}$ and over 10 times as much manganese. And meal #2 contains essential fatty acids, which aren't even present in the first meal.

The second meal is lacking in a few things provided by the first meal. Carcinogenic nitrites, THBQ, bromate and other dangerous additives are not present.

This comparison is just to show you the difference between two meals and to show you how important small changes in diet can be. Not getting vitamins in your meals and consuming chemical additives causes fatigue. Things in your diet, which you consume on a regular basis, may be undermining your health and making you tired.

This is just a simple and obvious comparison made between two meals that are available in any supermarket. The differences between the meals is important, because the lack of vitamins and minerals in meals like #1, and the burden of eating chemically laden food places on your liver, cause fatigue.

There is no need to worry about the issues of vegetarianism, organic produce, food combining whether or not dairy products should be consumed or other more sweeping changes you could make to your diet—if you are still consuming food that is full of additives and devoid of vitamins, like the food in the first lunch.

You don't need to become some sort of fanatic. It may seem to you that the world is divided into two camps. One camp has the health "nuts": people wearing Birkenstocks and tie-dyed prints, driving Volvos and lecturing you about this additive and that chemical. They always seem to be eating some amorphous congealed mass, purchased in a health food store and tasting like something you once smelled on a farm. The other camp is the "screw it, I'm going to die anyway" crowd, stuffing their faces with Coke and Cheetos. Don't feel pressured, and don't feel that you have to go off the deep end and start eating things that smell like a farm animal had it first. Just begin to make healthy decisions. You can eat normal food; just wean yourself from packaged and processed foods.

You do not have to disrupt your lifestyle to eat better. You can still enjoy a meal of a sandwich and a salad, but what a world of difference if you take a little time and pay attention to the quality of your food. Increasing the amount of nutrients and decreasing the sugar and added chemicals you get in your food will improve your health. Get the most food value out of each meal you eat and you will have incredible energy. Increasing the amount of nutrients and decreasing the sugar and added chemicals will improve your health.

Chemicals and additives drain your energy. The constant chemical bombarding you get with additives, chemicals and pesticides causes fatigue and can eventually lead to allergies and immune system problems. Considering the fact that everything that takes place in your body involves chemical reactions, it should be obvious that introducing chemicals to your body that do not belong there can have far-reaching implications to your health and energy. Denying the body vitamins and minerals by eating food that is nutrient-deficient undermines health. In order to survive, the body must conserve energy. It becomes fatigued.

Patients who eat nutrient-deficient, additive and sugar-loaded diets are continually asking questions like, "Doc, do you think that taking bee pollen will give me more energy?" It's how we're trained to think of health care: I can do anything to my body that I want to as long as I find the right pill to make me feel better. Unfortunately, that is a poor strategy for maintaining your health and energy.

If you are fatigued, the very first place you need to look is in your diet. This is like checking for gas if your car doesn't start. It is basic. No exotic herb, no medical regimen, not even extract from humming bird testicles will work if you do not have good nutrition.

Go on a caveman diet. This doesn't mean that you have to eat brontosaurus steaks and pterodactyl eggs. You don't have to go to the snack bar at Jurassic Park. Simply eat foods that were available 10,000 years ago. If the food comes in a bottle, box or a can, avoid it. Stop eating refined foods and those with chemical additives. Drink plenty of water. Get plenty of rest.

If your car doesn't function, you look at the simple, basic things—the battery, gas, whether or not it is in drive, before you pull out the engine and have it overhauled. This the way it should be with your body. Good nutrition is not an alternative therapy, like many doctors would have you believe. It is a fundamental part of good health.

Good nutrition is especially important considering the changes in agriculture over the past 100 years. The use of chemical fertilizers depletes the soil of trace nutrients like zinc, molybdenum, manganese and other minerals. A vegetable will not contain anything that is not in the soil that grows it. Chemical fertilizers enable farmers to grow large, attractive produce that has very little food value. Who hasn't taken a bite out of a nice, big, bright red apple only to find that it tastes like Styrofoam?

One hundred years ago, fewer than 3% of all deaths were from cancer. Today, one in four American men and one in five American women die of cancer. According to the National Cancer Institute, between 1950 and 1985 cancer in children increased 32%; bladder cancer increased 51%; testicular cancer increased 81%; kidney and renal pelvis cancer increased 82%; and non-Hodgkin's lymphoma (linked with pesticide exposure) increased by 123%. Much of this increase in cancer can be attributed to food additives and pesticides and is compounded by the fact that much of our food is depleted of vitamins. As more of the population becomes aware of the danger of chemicals, it is becoming increasingly popular to buy pesticide-free, organic produce.

If you do not have enough energy, it is important to pay attention to the quality of your food. You need to eat whole foods that are high in nutrition. You need to avoid additives and other chemicals as much as possible.

Chemicals cause fatigue. If you have ever had a hangover, you know the effect chemicals can have on you. A hangover is simply a state of chemical toxicity. Your fatigue may be due to a chemical "hangover."

## FAT

In the midst of the chemical onslaught your body goes through, the chief dietary villain the media and the medical profession have chosen is fat. People are eating turkey bologna and salami, loaded with cancer-causing nitrites, with a secure feeling that they are eating properly. Such products advertise that they are low in fat, and people who eat them sincerely believe that they are eating healthily.

Other products that advertise being low-fat are loaded with chemicals. Consider the low-fat dressing a few pages back. Low-fat doesn't automatically mean healthy. Actually the word *lite* is an ancient Sanskrit word meaning: "full of chemicals."

The food pyramid, designed to replace the now-defunct four food groups, makes no distinction between refined and whole grains. People are being taught that grain products are low in fat and good for them. As a result, they are consuming tons of white, refined noodles, breads and other nutrient-deficient, chemically laden products, thinking that they are eating healthily.

Fat is not the unmixed evil that many experts would have you believe. In fact, many people who suffer from fatigue are on low-fat diets.

If your fat consumption is too low, you will not absorb oil-soluble nutrients very well. You become deficient in essential fatty acids, vitamin A, vitamin E, vitamin K and possibly vitamin D. Fat is necessary for the proper functioning of the endocrine system. Cholesterol is necessary for production of adrenal hormones.

Deficiencies in oil-soluble nutrients can affect the skin, the musculoskeletal system, the endocrine system and the immune system. If your diet is too low in fat, you may experience fatigue, dry skin, frequent colds, frequent bladder infections, menstrual problems, allergies, muscle fatigability and even tension headaches.

Dr. Pritikin, and recently, Dr. Dean Ornish, have had success with heart patients by putting them on a 10% fat diet. Their success has many erroneously believing that we all need to be on a 10% fat diet. Actually, a diet this low in fat is a medical treatment meant to be used in extreme cases. It is, in itself, an extreme measure.

Dr. Ornish has a program that decreases plaque in arteries as well as reducing cholesterol. His diet only allows 10% fat and the patient must do deep breathing, exercise and stress reduction techniques. One very interesting thing about Dr. Ornish's program is that the low-fat diet is not particularly effective without the exercise and stress reduction components.

Some people do well on low-fat diets because some of the worst foods in their diets are fats. Animals are at the top of the food chain. Insecticides permeate everything in the environment, including water and vegetation. Animals consume water and vegetation and store the chemicals in their fat. Over time, the chemicals in the animals' tissue become more concentrated.

Butter and cheese are very high in pesticide residues. The FDA tested cheddar cheese from around the nation and found 100 pesticide and industrial chemical residues in the samples. These included BHC, DDT, dieldrin, heptachlor, HCB and octachlor, which were found in 25% of the samples.

Fatty foods potentiate carcinogenic effects of the chemicals in the food. In other words, if you consume chemicals in the presence of fat, the chemicals are more dangerous.

Less than 1% of all meat is tested for carcinogens. In 1988, an internal audit by the inspector general's office of the USDA discovered that tainted meat had been sold for consumption, even after federal inspectors found that it was chemically contaminated.

Meat and dairy products not only have chemicals from the environment, they have chemicals that are purposely given to the animals by the farmers. Farmers purchase half of all the antibiotics sold in this country. They are added to animal feed, indiscriminately, at the discretion of the farmer.

Dairy cows are now being given bovine growth hormone, or BGH. The manufacturer prefers it to be called bovine somatotrophin. (Bovine somatotrophin is a less-threatening name—better marketing. Of course that would make the acronym BS, which probably is more appropriate.) The FDA has given farmers permission to use BGH *without having to tell consumers.*

The FDA justifies this lack of consumer information by telling the public that BGH isn't found in the milk. Of course, nothing is said about BGH undermining the animals' health, making it necessary for the farmer to give more antibiotics and other drugs that will find their way into the milk. Even if BGH were totally harmless, as the FDA claims, there have been enough outcries from consumers to justify labeling.

In general, there is always the possibility that meat and dairy products contain chemicals. A lot of the problem has to do with how the animals are raised. Hog barns are built with slatted floors, over large pits where the excrement is collected below. The hogs are in tiny stalls and inhale the fumes of their own waste, 24 hours a day. The hogs are never allowed outside. Because of the crowded, filthy conditions, pneumonia is always a threat.

In order to prevent pneumonia, drugs are given to the hogs. Sulfa drugs are very popular among hog farmers because they are cheap. One of the more popular drugs is sulfanethazine, which has been linked to thyroid problems in humans and is a possible carcinogen. Ten percent of the slaughtered hogs tested (remember that only 1% of all animals are tested), have sulfamethazine residues. Sulfamethazine is only one chemical. Animal fat has a lot of chemicals in it. It is wise to reduce your consumption of it.

Not all fat is created equal. It is important for you to understand the difference between fats. Vegetable oils, raw nuts and avocados are sources of good fat and should not be completely shunned. Some kinds of fat should be avoided, but not all. If you are careful about the quality of the fat you eat, you can eat a diet that is higher in fat. Some sources of fat follow:

*Meat and dairy:* High in saturated fat and high in chemicals. There is wisdom in eating poultry and fish, which are low in fat, and selecting low-fat cuts of meat. You can buy organically grown meat, free range chickens and dairy products from cows that have not been given antibiotics. If you eat animal products, it is wise to find animals that have not been fed steroids or antibiotics, and animals that have not been raised on factory-farms that abuse them and put out an unhealthy product.

*Vegetable oils:* Around 1900, all salad oil was produced by pressing flax seeds. This oil was very high in essential fatty acids. Now most oils are extracted with heat or chemicals. Once an oil has been heated, it has absolutely no nutritional value. It may even be toxic. You should stay away from oils that have been heat or chemically extracted and buy only cold-pressed oils. If the oil is in a clear bottle, exposed to light, you should not consume it. The naturally obtained oils are not stored this way because they can become rancid. If the oil is in a clear bottle, exposed to light, it probably was extracted with heat or chemicals.

Heat damages oil and potentially makes it carcinogenic. This is why you should never eat deep-fried foods. It's okay to sauté foods in olive oil. Never reheat or reuse oil.

Olive oil is relatively stable to heat. You can sauté food in olive oil and not worry too much about it being toxic. There are different grades of olive oil. The highest quality imported olive oil is graded as extra virgin. The next highest quality is virgin, which is between 1.0 and 3.3 percent acid. Olive oil which has been graded as *pure* is the lowest grade of olive oil, because the producers thought it would be better than grading it as *crappy*, which would be bad for sales. It's the same reason you can't buy a "small" soda pop or popcorn at the movies. Olive oil grades are a lot like going to the snack bar at the movies and the soda pop comes in three sizes: large, extra large and jumbo. Pure olive oil has a high acid content, which has been neutralized with chemicals; it is not of acceptable quality. Domestic olive oil has three grades: virgin—the first pressing and highest American grade of olive oil; refined—second pressing which has added chemicals to neutralize the acidity and refined olive residue oil—good for crankcases or to substitute at a "Wesson" party. When buying olive oil, look for the words *virgin* or *extra virgin* on the label.

***Hydrogenated or partially hydrogenated oil:*** Avoid these like the plague. They are implicated in heart disease. They interfere with normal fat metabolism. They stay in the body for a very long time. Hydrogenation is a way of artificially saturating an unsaturated fat. This makes an oil into a solid and makes it ship and store better. Margarine and mayonnaise are made with hydrogenated oils. Hydrogenated and partially hydrogenated oils are found in a lot of packaged and convenience foods.

***Avocados and nuts:*** These are excellent sources of oil-soluble nutrients. Make sure that the nuts are raw; do not eat roasted nuts. Peanut butter, cashew butter, almond butter and tahinni are very nutritious, but get the organic version. Smooth commercial peanut butters have added sugar, hydrogenated oil and other chemicals. Buy peanut butter that has the oil separate from the rest of the peanut butter, like Smuckers and Holsum. If you read the label of these products, you will see that they only have peanuts and salt.

***Deep fried foods:*** Carcinogenic empty calories. Avoid them.

Eating the wrong kinds of fat can undermine your health and sap your energy. Just make sure that you eat fat, even good fats, in moderation.

## CARBOHYDRATES

The popularity of low-fat diets is beginning to wane. Carbohydrates are the new villains. Low- (or no-) carbohydrate diets, like the Atkins diet, have become very popular. We have found that insulin makes you fat, but instead of eating healthy foods in all three categories, carbohydrate, fat and protein, we condemn an entire food group. Carcinogenic and otherwise unhealthy foods are okay; eat all of the butter, sausage, hydrogenated oils and chemicals that you want, just stay away from carbohydrates. Do you see a pattern here? When health professionals begin to notice kidney problems and other health problems from eating too much fat and protein, then protein will be condemned and a new guru with a different simplistic, idiotic approach to nutrition will appear.

One of the reasons these low- or no-carbohydrate diets seem to be so good is the fact that Americans eat far too many refined carbohydrates. When they stop eating refined carbohydrates, even if the diet that they change to is less than ideal, they lose weight and feel better.

Carbohydrate intolerance, or hyper-insulinism, may be worth mentioning here. Patients who are carbohydrate intolerant may suffer from fatigue, poor concentration, low blood sugar, intestinal bloating, increased fat storage (especially pot belly or large buttocks), increased blood pressure and depression.

Some doctors use the following test to find if carbohydrate intolerance is a problem. If you try this test, find a doctor to monitor your progress with this test. For two weeks the patient does not eat any carbohydrate, except for a piece of 100% whole grain bread at breakfast. They eat no products that contain grain such as bread, rolls, rice oatmeal, pasta, pancakes, cereal and muffins. They eat no sweets, including products that contain sugar like ketchup and other condiments. Fruit and fruit juice is avoided as are potatoes, corn and beans. Milk and yogurt are not allowed.

Meat is permitted (except for cold cuts), poultry, fish, eggs, cheese and any vegetables (except for corn, potatoes and beans). The patient should also eat as much food as desired. This is only for two weeks, but it must be the full two weeks without breaking discipline.

If, after two weeks on the program, the patient has lost weight, improved his or her mood, began bloating less or has other significant improvements in health and well-being, the patient probably needs to be eating fewer carbohydrates. After the two-week test, gradually add carbohydrates to the diet. No sugar or refined carbohydrates are allowed. A potato or a serving of beans is added. The patient sees how he or she feels for the next couple of days. If symptoms do not return, carbohydrate intake can be increased a little more.

If symptoms return at some point after the increase in carbohydrate intake, it's been increased too much. It needs to be reduced it again. The patient can experiment with the diet and find the ideal amount of carbohydrate consumption. As health improves, so should the tolerance for carbohydrates. This is especially true if yeast is a factor.

The test may be a little extreme; there is likelihood that it will cause ketosis. Ketones are a by product of fat breaking down. High levels of ketones create ketosis, which is stressful on the body. Simply reducing carbohydrate consumption, or going on a more reasonable diet, like *Sugar Busters* may accomplish the same weight loss and increase in energy. The test is worth mentioning here because so many people go on the Atkins diet and say, "It's the best I've ever felt in my life." In all likelihood they are carbohydrate intolerant (thinking of this situation as insulin insensitivity might be better).

## Vegetarianism

It is not necessary to become a vegetarian to become thin and healthy. There are, however, some health advantages to vegetarian eating. Vegetarians usually have less fat and fewer chemicals in their diet. The vegetarian diet is easier to digest than a diet that contains meat and dairy. As a rule, vegetarian meals are usually much lower in calories than meals containing animal products.

While it is not absolutely necessary that you become a vegetarian, it would be helpful if you changed how you think about food. Most Americans don't think a meal is complete without meat. In many other cultures beans and bread is a meal. In this country they are an appetizer, snack or side dish.

Vegetarians often suffer from fatigue, especially salad bar vegetarians who live on iceberg lettuce and bread. Many vegetarians eat a lot of refined food. Nutrient deficiency is a problem for many of them. It's not that the vegetarian diet is inherently low in certain nutrients; it's just that people who eat meat get certain vitamins easier than vegetarians do.

Many vegetarians are deficient in vitamin $B_{12}$, which is a nutrient that is in meat and dairy products. Vegetarians can get it from their intestinal bacteria, but good bowel health is necessary for this. If a vegetarian's bowel is not healthy, he or she may be deficient in $B_{12}$. A deficiency in $B_{12}$ can cause fatigue, depression, and poor concentration among other things, and supplementation is usually necessary for vegetarians.

Many argue that the vegetarians tend to be protein deficient because the protein available to them is not as complete as animal protein. A complete protein is one that contains all eight essential amino acids. An essential amino acid is one that the body cannot manufacture; it must be eaten in the diet. Animal proteins tend to have all eight essential amino acids. Most vegetables do not have complete proteins. They may have some of the essential amino acids, but not all of them. A vegetarian usually has to eat more than one food to get a complete protein. If you eat a whole grain and a legume (bean, pea or nut), you get the same quality protein as a steak. Quinoa, a grain, is also a complete protein.

Many people become vegetarians because they don't digest meat well or because eating meat doesn't make them feel very good. This is may be due to the stomach not producing enough hydrochloric acid. These people tend to live on starch and leafy vegetables, because these foods seem easier to digest. Fatigue, due to a deficiency of essential amino acids, vitamin $B_{12}$ and many minerals, is often a problem. Supplementation may be necessary. Vitamin $B_{12}$ deficiency is a common source of fatigue in vegetarians. Taking vitamin $B_{12}$, a multimineral and an amino acid supplement (containing all eight of the essential amino acids) often gives these people incredible energy.

In nonvegetarians, vitamin $B_{12}$ deficiency is due to a problem absorbing the vitamin. As people get older, stomach hydrochloric acid production decreases, as does $B_{12}$ absorption. Older people tend to eat less meat and dairy because of their digestion. $B_{12}$ deficiency is the most common cause of fatigue and depression in older people. Sometimes the deficiency is so severe that the individual develops symptoms that mimic Alzheimer's disease. Often the blood test for $B_{12}$ is normal, but the patient is still deficient. (A health care provider trained in nutrition can help you determine if $B_{12}$ deficiency is an issue for you.)

Since $B_{12}$ deficiency usually exists because of an absorption problem, it is commonly treated with $B_{12}$ injections. Oral $B_{12}$ is effective if the dosage is high enough (more than one or two milligrams per day); also using a sublingual $B_{12}$ (like $B_{12}$-2000 lozenges by Biotics Research) is very well-absorbed. Also it is a good idea to take folic acid when taking $B_{12}$. ($B_{12}$-2000 contains 800 mcg. of folic acid.)

## Confusion About Diets

People are so confused about what they should and should not eat. There is so much conflicting information about diet. Registered dieticians talk about the food pyramid, which would give you a diet heavy in grains. Dr. Atkins talks about carbohydrates as being the source of all our health woes. Dr. Dean Ornish and Covert Bailey decry the evils of fat. John Robbins makes a strong case for a totally vegan diet. The Zone diet seeks to give a balance between protein, carbohydrate and fat. *Sugar Busters* seeks to reduce insulin production. A lot of the information seems to be conflicting and the various dietary gurus have harsh things to say about each other's diets.

None of the dietary experts can dispute the nutritional rules below. They may offer refinements like, "Watch your fat consumption," "Watch your carbohydrate consumption" or "Stay away from animal products," but none of the experts would say there is anything wrong with the following list of dietary advice. There may also be a little controversy about the implications of not following the advice. (Some may dispute that sugar consumption will cause yeast to grow in the intestines, for example, but they would not dispute that consumption of refined sugar is a bad thing.) The advice about water has become controversial, but drinking a lot of water isn't a problem if you are not drinking a lot of coffee, tea, sodas or other drinks.

## BASIC DIET

*1. Drink at least eight 8oz glasses of water each day:* You need water to keep your cells hydrated and protected, to eliminate waste and ensure the health of your mucus membranes. Adequate hydration will improve a number of health problems including sinusitis, constipation, inflammation, allergies, fatigue, joint pain, headaches and many other afflictions.

Your body cannot adequately eliminate waste products without enough water. If toxic chemicals or heavy metal poisoning is at the root of your health problems you will have a much easier time getting better when you are properly hydrated.

*2. Eat plenty of vegetables:* Plenty means that at least _ to _ of the food you eat (by volume). Vegetables are very high in fiber, vitamin C, folic acid and minerals. They provide you with many health benefits, such as the following:

- Fiber in vegetables slows the absorption of fat and toxins. One of the best ways to lose weight is to eat plenty of fiber. Eating adequate fiber can help normalize cholesterol levels and blood pressure.
- Vegetables nourish normal flora, which in turn nourish the lining of the GI tract, produce vitamins and inhibit yeast and other undesirable organisms.
- Vegetables speed up bowel transit time, which reduces bowel toxicity and prevents irritation of the GI lining.
- Vegetables contain folic acid, which is necessary to produce serotonin (preventing

depression and overeating), increases energy and helps reduce the chances for a heart attack.

- The minerals in vegetables help prevent osteoporosis. (Other nutrients besides calcium are important for healthy bone.) Minerals are also important enzyme cofactors, so most major functions of the body are dependent on minerals.
- Eating vegetables can reduce the instance of cancer and heart disease, increase your energy and mental clarity, reduce the problems caused by bowel and liver toxicity, help reduce the symptoms of allergies, asthma, arthritis, skin problems, digestive problems, sinusitis, chronic pain and many other health problems.
- Eating vegetables helps to alkalize the diet. (We will go into the concept of alkaline and acid ash foods in the next section.)

Ideally $\frac{1}{2}$ to $\frac{3}{4}$ of the volume of the food you eat should be vegetables. Corn and potatoes don't count as vegetables. Fruit is also good for you; it is a good source of vitamin C and fiber. Eating vegetables is stressed here because when people are told to eat more fruits and vegetables, they tend to increase fruit intake but not vegetable intake.

*3. Avoid deep fried food, partially hydrogenated oil and hydrogenated oil:* As time passes, we keep finding more bad things about hydrogenated oil and fried foods. Hydrogenation is the food industry's way of turning a liquid oil into a solid fat. This gives packaged foods a longer shelf life than if they were made with natural oils. Hydrogenation produces trans fats, which have been linked to a number of health problems such as the following:

- Cancer: Women with higher levels of trans fats in their cells are much more likely to develop breast cancer than women with low levels of trans fats.
- Pain and inflammation become much worse for patients who consume hydrogenated oils. They chemically prevent the formation of natural anti-inflammatory substances that are normally produced by the body. If you suffer from chronic pain or have recently been injured, strictly avoid hydrogenated oil.
- Heart disease: High levels of trans fats create platelet aggregation, which is the beginning of the plaque associated with coronary heart disease. Lately a lot has been written linking inflammation with heart disease.
- Trans fats are incorporated into the cells and make them less resistant to chemicals, bacteria and viruses. This could be a source of immune system problems.
- There may be a link between trans fats and ADD, depression and fatigue. Brain and nerve tissue have a high content of fat. Some researches believe that when trans fats are incorporated into the nerve cells they affect function creating problems like ADD and depression.
- Muscle fatigue and skin problems are also linked to hydrogenated oils.

Most chips and fried snacks contain hydrogenated oils. Hydrogenated oils are found in a lot of packaged foods like crackers, cereals and even bread. They are in margarine (margarine is much worse for you than butter), mayonnaise and a lot of bottled salad dressings. Read labels.

Not all fats are bad for you. Permissible fats include raw nuts (not roasted), virgin or extra virgin olive oil and avocados.

*4. Avoid refined sugar:* The average American eats 150 pounds of refined sugar per year. Compare that to seven pounds per year consumed in England in 1750. Refined sugar increases insulin and adrenal hormone production and can cause the following health problems.

- Increased production of adrenal hormones causes the body to excrete essential minerals.
- Sugar consumption increases the body's need for vitamins B & C.
- Eating a lot of sugar aggravates many of the problems we associate with emotional stress. Sugar stresses the adrenal glands.
- Sugar feeds yeast and other one-celled organisms found in the bowel, causing them to multiply. These organisms produce toxins, irritate the lining of the GI tract and take the place of normal, more beneficial flora, thus removing the benefits of helpful bacteria.
- Eating sugar causes blood sugar swings. Blood sugar increases immediately after consuming sugar, prompting the body to produce insulin. Excess insulin creates more sugar cravings. More sugar is eaten, more insulin produced, etc. This stresses the pancreas and sets the stage for adult-onset diabetes.
- There is a connection between sugar consumption and high cholesterol. Patients with Syndrome X (high cholesterol, high LDL, low HDL and high triglycerides) often have the problem because of

consumption of sugar and refined carbohydrates.
- Sugar consumption can make pain and inflammation worse.
- Sugar can cause or aggravate allergies, sinusitis, asthma, irritable bowel, Candidiasis, migraine headaches, fatigue, depression and even heart disease.

**5. *Avoid refined carbohydrates:*** The average American gets 50% of his or her calories from refined carbohydrates. Refined carbohydrates are grains that have had the fiber, vitamin E, B vitamins, bran and germ removed. In other words, the nutrients have been removed and you are left with the starch. They create all of the same health problems created by refined sugar. Go back and read the problems caused by refined sugar and realize that the list is exactly the same for refined starches

Refined carbohydrates fill you up—but not with vitamins and minerals. This stresses your digestive system and your endocrine system. Eating refined carbohydrates uses up precious vitamins and minerals.

Often people eat refined carbohydrates because they are low in fat and mistakenly think that because they are "complex carbohydrates" that they are actually good for you.    Refined carbohydrates include white bread, white rice, and pasta that are not labeled *whole grain*. Read the labels on bread. Brown-colored bread labeled *wheat bread* isn't usually whole wheat. If the label says *enriched, white flour* on it, you're not getting a whole grain. Use brown rice instead of white rice.

**6. *Avoid chemical additives:*** Avoid processed foods and chemicals. The average American consumes 10 pounds of chemical additives every year. This has had a devastating effect on our health. The FDA tests single additives, but no one has any idea what combinations of additives do to us. Stay away from packaged foods with chemical additives and you will be much healthier.

**7. *Eat slowly, chew your food thoroughly:*** Ideally, chew your food until it is liquid. You will be satisfied with less food and you will have better digestion. Your saliva has enzymes that facilitate digestion. Also, it is easier to digest small particles than large ones. Most people eat too fast. Not chewing well stresses your digestive system and can lead to poor absorption of nutrients, digestive problems like gas and bloating and promote the growth of harmful bacteria in the digestive tract.

**8. *Never skip meals:*** Skipping meals stresses your adrenal glands. If you are trying to lose weight, not eating is a poor strategy because your metabolism will slow down to accommodate the reduction in calories. As a result you become fatigued and will ultimately gain weight.

### Alkaline Ash Diet

Having given you a list of noncontroversial ways to improve your diet, let's add one controversial subject, the alkaline ash diet. I hope it does not add to your confusion, but people who follow the concepts you are about to read really seem to enjoy better health than people who do not.

Proponents of the alkaline ash diet believe that we eat too many acid-forming foods and that excess acid is a source of many of our chronic illnesses. Critics of the diet say that the body's pH is tightly regulated and cannot be affected by subtle changes in diet. What the critics do not say is that they tried putting chronically ill people on the diet and did not see good results. You won't hear critics say this because the opposite is true. People who go on this diet usually are rewarded with better health. This diet is appropriate and beneficial for just about any chronic health problem.

The critics may be right about the diet directly affecting pH. In all likelihood the diet probably affects the body's ability to buffer acids. In other words, the "acid" diet probably doesn't change the pH of the body but rather makes the body work harder to maintain its pH.

According to proponents of this diet, eating the wrong foods creates acid systemically. Diets that are high in fat, protein and simple sugars are too acid. To reduce the acid burden the body links acids with alkaline minerals (like potassium, calcium and magnesium) and excretes them.

The excess acid load has a negative effect on energy production in the cells, enzyme function and tissue resilience and repair. This acid burden, when coupled with constant exposure to pollution, food additives, and poor digestion, burdens the immune system and exceeds the body's reserves. A continuous state of distress can emerge, resulting in the increase of the chemical messengers of distress (such as cortisol, adrenaline, and insulin).

People like Dr. Carey Reams, Edgar Cayce and others recommend the ideas behind the diet. Dr. Reams was an agricultural biochemist. He called his technique, The Reams Biological Theory of Ionization. He had adapted a soil and plant testing technique to test urine and saliva. His test consisted of seven parameters: sugar brix, urine pH, saliva pH, conductivity, cell debris, nitrate nitrogen and ammonia nitrogen. It was accomplished by using laboratory instruments and techniques normally used for agricultural testing.

Dr. Reams believed that we don't live off the food that we eat; we live off the energy in the food we eat. He believed that it is better to eat live, raw foods than it is to eat cooked foods. Some confusion in terminology has resulted because of the way that the discussion evolved. In investigating how different foods might affect the acid-alkaline balance, various foods were burned to ash in the laboratory, and the pH of the resulting ash was measured. These foods were then classified as acid, alkaline or neutral ash foods.

In fact, if you read various authors about the alkaline ash diet you will see lots of inconsistencies. One author will say that nuts are all acid; another will say the almonds and cashews are alkaline. Quinoa is either acid or alkaline depending on who you read. There are differences in opinion about how pH should be measured. One author will say the urine should be pH 7, another will say that a pH of 6.8 is good.

Various alternative practitioners have referred to acid- and alkaline-forming foods, based on the reaction of foods in the body. One thing that is considered a highly acidic way to eat is the combining of carbohydrate with protein.

In general, alkaline ash foods contain more magnesium, calcium, potassium and/or sodium. These are minerals that form alkaline compounds. Most fruits and vegetables are considered alkaline. Acid ash foods contain more chloride, phosphorus or sulphur, minerals that form acid compounds. These acid ash foods include meat, fish, poultry, legumes and grains, which all contain high levels of phosphorus, and mustard and eggs, which contain sulphur. Some fruits like plums, prunes, cranberries or rhubarb are considered acid-forming since they contain either oxalic or benzoic acid, organic acids which are not completely broken down in the body.

There is some individual variation as to whether foods are treated as alkaline or as acid. Genetics also plays a role; some groups can handle protein better than others. One possible explanation may be that people of different blood types handle protein differently. People who are blood type O seem to do better with more protein. Many groups of people who have not been exposed to civilization and therefore enjoy life relatively free of our civilized chronic degenerative diseases eat a diet that is a little more acidic (according to the model presented) than what is recommended here. Their diets are very nutrient-dense and that is at least as important as pH balance.

For regaining health, eating 80% alkaline foods and 20% acid foods has been recommended. Eating four vegetables and two fruits to one starchy food and one protein food approximates this number. The reason this proportion works well here is that most Americans eat a high-acid diet. We eat a lot of grain and protein and not a lot of vegetables. We also tend to combine starch and protein. Changing these eating patterns often has dramatic results in improving health.

The excess acid load has a negative effect on energy production in the cells, enzyme function and tissue resilience and repair. This acid burden when coupled with constant exposure to pollution, food additives and poor digestion burdens the immune system and exceeds the body's reserves. A continuous state of distress can emerge, resulting in the increase of the chemical messengers of distress (such as cortisol, adrenaline and insulin).

Whether or not you believe in the effect that food can have on your systemic pH, the alkaline ash diet is a very healthy way to eat. In fact, the issue may be more about our capacity to buffer acids or alkaline foods. A diet that is too high in protein and refined foods may make it harder for you to regulate pH; it doesn't put you in acidosis. Blood never becomes acidic during life; the critics of this way of thinking are right about that. The diet is, however, effective for restoring health—for whatever reason. Increase the amount of alkaline foods and decrease the amount of acid foods to help to restore your health.

There are those who have taken this information to mean that all acid foods are bad all of the time and that you should never eat animal products, and that all acid-forming foods are akin to poison.

There are some problems with this way of thinking; a diet in which these acid ash foods are absent can lead to deficiencies that undermine the body's ability to maintain the proper blood pH. Meat and other animal foods provide protein and vitamin $B_{12}$; red meats provide zinc. Both are needed for the regulation of acid-base balance. Fat-soluble vitamins and protein found in organ meats, shellfish and meat in general help maintain the health of the lungs and kidneys. Good lung and kidney function is necessary for good acid-base regulation.

The concept of alkaline and acid ash is a good one, but you also have to take into account the need to eat natural, nutrient-dense foods. Never forget that diet is individual and that one person's meat is another's poison. With that in mind, take a look at what kinds of foods improve alkalinity.

*Alkaline foods:* Fruit (most), vegetables (except peas, beans), lentils (some consider lentil acid, others consider them alkaline), spices, herbs and seasonings, seeds and nuts.
*Acid foods:* Meat, fish, poultry, eggs, grains and legumes.

This, of course, is a generality. Some grains, like wild rice, quinoa and oat are mildly alkaline. Quail eggs and duck eggs are mildly alkaline. Nuts are generally alkaline, but walnuts and Brazil nuts are acidic. There are books written on the alkaline diet, or you can ask your health care provider. In general, alkaline ash foods are those that contain large quantities of magnesium, calcium, potassium and/or sodium, minerals that form alkaline compounds. Most fruits and vegetables are considered alkaline. Acid ash foods are those that contain chloride, phosphorus or sulphur, minerals that form acid compounds. These acid ash foods include meat, fish, poultry, legumes and grains, which all contain high levels of phosphorus, and mustard and eggs, which contain sulphur.

Many foods that seem acidic to us are actually alkaline. Foods like lemons, oranges, and tomatoes, for example, are considered alkaline.

It must be stressed that these lists vary and sometimes it is best to follow the general rules: grains and proteins are acid, and fruits, nuts, seeds and vegetables are alkaline. The important thing to do is to eat a lot of produce and to eat whole and unprocessed foods (like the advice given in the Basic Diet).

If you want to restore your health, about 80% of your diet should be alkaline foods. In more practical terms, the recommendation was four vegetables and two fruits to one starchy food and one protein food. This is the proportion of foods for the day. If, for instance, you have 3 oz. of protein one day, you need 12 oz. of vegetables and 8 oz. of fruit for the day. You are also allowed 3 oz. of grain, but it is not to be eaten with the meat.

Maintaining health is easier. If you do not have any major health problems, you need to eat 60% alkaline foods to maintain your health. This translates to one protein, one starch, two vegetables and one fruit. If you have 6 oz. of protein, you then need 12 oz. of vegetable and 6 oz. of fruit for the day. You are also allowed 6 oz of grain—but it is not to be eaten with the meat. When you eat this way, fruits and vegetables will dominate your diet; if these are fresh and raw, so much the better. If you can get organic produce, that will remove the burden that pesticides place on your body. There is a fair amount of variation in what is considered alkaline and what is considered acid. For that reason, we are going to try to avoid all of the controversy and make it simpler.

Animal products are on the list of acid foods, but you are allowed some of these—unlike those eating a strict vegetarian diet, you can have some meat. It's like following Thomas Jefferson's advice to use meat as a condiment, which may be healthier than a strict vegetarian diet.

Grains are on the list of foods that should be minimally consumed. What do Americans eat? They eat sandwiches, chicken and rice, meat and potatoes and other combinations of meat and starch, in other words, an extremely acid-forming diet. Eat more alkaline foods and fewer acid foods and your energy will increase and your health will improve.

Americans tend to eat a lot of grains. Grains are considered acidic and we probably eat more than are healthy for us. Limiting grain consumption may be a good idea. Many patients do better when they limit or eliminate grains.

If you need more energy or if you have *any* chronic health problems you need to follow the proceeding diet. Even though there is a lot of controversy about the alkaline ash diet (even among proponents who can't seem to agree on particulars), patients do very well when they follow it. There are a few controversial concepts added to the Basic Diet like food combining and alkaline ash eating, but try it. This diet does seem to help a lot of health problems.

## HEALING DIET

1. Drink at least eight (8) ounce glasses of water each day.
2. Eat plenty of vegetables.
3. Avoid deep fried food, partially hydrogenated oil and hydrogenated oil.
4. Avoid refined sugar.
5. Avoid refined carbohydrates.
6. Avoid chemical additives.

7.  Eat slowly, and chew your food thoroughly.
8.  Never skip meals.
9.  Follow the rules for more alkaline eating. These include the following:

- If you have any chronic health problems eat 80% alkaline ash foods and 20% acid ash foods. In more practical terms, eat four vegetables and two fruits to one starchy food and one protein food.
- If you enjoy good health, maintain it by eating 60% alkaline ash foods and 40% acid ash foods.
- Eat mostly *raw* produce. It is okay to eat cooked food, but we are going to follow Dr. Reams' idea that we don't live off the food that we eat, we live off the energy in the food we eat. It is better to eat live, raw foods than it is to eat cooked foods.
- Do not eat protein and carbohydrate together—this acts to acidify the body.
- Do not eat fruit with grains or other foods—this acts to acidify the body.
- Realize that alcohol and caffeine are extremely acidic and should be limited.

When you follow the basic diet you are still able to follow familiar eating patterns. You can have meat and potatoes, a sandwich made with protein and a whole grain bread or fruit in your oatmeal. Adding the disciplines of the alkaline ash diet may make it so you have to change how you think about eating. You really have to just think of eating as providing your body with fuel and not about likes and dislikes. You will probably have to plan your meals in advance and not just grab food on the run. Try it very strictly for 30 days. Most people can do anything for 30 days. It will improve your health and energy and help you to see the connection between how you eat and how you feel.

Because eating this way is so different, here are some daily menu suggestions.

| Day 1: | Breakfast | Apple with almond butter |
|--------|-----------|--------------------------|
| | Lunch | Tuna (mix it with olive oil chopped onion and celery); celery stalks, carrot sticks or cucumber slices |
| | Dinner | Sweet potato (you can use some clarified butter, which is alkaline), large green salad (oil and cider vinegar) and mixed, cooked vegetables |
| | Snack | Any fruit, nuts or any vegetable |
| Day 2: | Breakfast | Oatmeal |
| | Lunch | Turkey, large green salad |
| | Dinner | Brown rice, cooked vegetables, large green salad |
| | Snack | Any fruit, nuts or any vegetable |
| Day 3 | Breakfast | Quinoa |
| | Lunch | Chicken vegetable soup, large green salad |
| | Dinner | Chicken, large green salad, cooked vegetables |
| | Snack | Any fruit, nuts or any vegetable |
| Day 4: | Breakfast | Melon |
| | Lunch | Hommus, taboule, goat feta cheese and cucumber slices |
| | Dinner | Beef vegetable soup, large green salad |
| | Snack | Any fruit, nuts or any vegetable. |
| Day 5: | Breakfast | Vegetable omelet (chopped onion, spinach, tomatoes and bell peppers [if nightshades are not a problem for you]) |
| | Lunch | Stir fried vegetables and brown rice |
| | Dinner | Broiled salmon, avocado and a green salad |

See the appendix for recipes and ideas for soups, salads and juices. Try to dominate your diet with raw foods. If your meals have a lot of cooked food, snack on raw vegetables. Another way to get raw, alkaline food in the diet is to make fresh vegetable juice; see the appendix. If you are busy, simply eating protein with a lot of vegetables is a quick, easy way to make a meal. For example, you can broil a chicken breast, boil some broccoli and make a large salad. It's fast and it's fairly alkaline. Another strategy for busy people is to make stews or soups and eat them throughout the week. Just snack on raw vegetables to make sure that you get enough raw food.

In restaurants, it isn't that difficult to eat a relatively alkaline meal. In an Italian restaurant you can order chicken, fish or meat with cooked vegetables and a large salad. Even at McDonalds you can take the bun off of your quarter pounder and order a salad. McDonalds even has a salad with chicken in it. Many fast food restaurants now have salad bars. In a Mexican restaurant you can order fajitas without the tortilla. In a Chinese or Thai restaurant you can get stir-fried vegetables with rice; you can also get a non-fried spring roll as an appetizer.

Raw foods are very good for you. There may be some validity to the argument that we consume the energy from the food we eat. Raw foods have enzymes and higher levels of vitamins like folic acid and vitamin C. Some people, however have problems when they eat a lot of raw vegetables. If you are such a person, call this to the attention of your health care practitioner. You may need nutritional support for the gall bladder (Beta-TCP, by Biotics Research helps thin bile). If someone pokes you under the right side of the ribcage, does it hurt; this may be an indication of problems with the gall bladder. You may need bile salts or you may need pancreatic enzymes.

## STRESS

Hans Selye conducted some experiments that today may have gotten animal rights activists upset (or at least gotten him a visit from the *Soys in the 'Hood*). Selye's assistant, Gunter, is credited with much of Selye's success by exercising a little damage control. He wisely convinced Hans to use rats for his experiments, instead of Selye's first choice, baby seals, and saved the project from being beset upon by PETA.

Thanks to Gunter, Selye conducted his experiments on rats, which hardly raised an eyebrow. No one seems to care if you experiment on an ugly animal. Of course it was the 1930s and this sort of thing was not as big of an issue as it is today.

The experiments involved creating stress in rats. Hans' early attempts at subjecting them to IRS audits were not very successful. Being a lab rat doesn't pay very well, and most of the animals were using the short form. Gunter again suggested some changes and saved the experiment. The rats were made to tread water with their legs tied until they became exhausted and died. Many humans would find this less stressful than dealing with the IRS, but it worked very well with the rats.

Dr. Selye took the rats at various stages of their ordeal and dissected out their adrenal glands. He found that the adrenal glands responded to stress in three distinct stages. In the initial stage, the adrenal glands enlarge and the blood supply to them increases. As the stress continues, the adrenal glands begin to shrink. Eventually, if the stress continues, the adrenal glands reach the third stage, which is adrenal exhaustion.

You may ask yourself, "What do rat adrenal glands have to do with me?" You may even be saying to yourself, "That's disgusting, what he did to the rats. How do I join the *Soys in the 'Hood*?" You may be thinking, "What's an adrenal gland?" You may even be thinking, "I'm tired. I think that I'll read this later."

If you are tired, or have other health problems, it may well have to do with your adrenal glands. The adrenal glands produce their hormones in response to stress. They are responsible for the fight or flight response. In a stressful situation, they make your blood pressure increase, transfer blood from your intestines to your extremities, increase your heart rate, suppress your immune system and increase your blood's clotting ability.

There is some new research that indicates that women respond differently to stress than men. For a woman, stress creates a change in brain chemistry that makes her want to bond with other women and tend to her children. This is new research, but look for new information from the scientific community on the difference between how men and women respond to stress.

The fight or flight response is meant to be short-lived. When primitive man walked through the forest, he'd see a saber-toothed tiger, which would really freak him out since saber-toothed tigers were supposed to have been extinct for thousands of years. His heart rate would increase; his pupils would dilate; his blood would go out of his digestive system and into his arms and legs; his blood-clotting ability would improve; he would become more aware and his blood pressure would rise. At that point he'd either pick up a stick and try to fight the animal or run like hell to go find a veterinary orthodontist (I guess the new research indicates that if a woman saw the tiger, she'd find another woman, have some tea and coffee cake and talk about it). The physiological changes brought on by the adrenal glands would make the body more efficient at doing either of those things. It is called the fight or flight response.

If our primitive man survived the ordeal, chances are it would be a while before such a strain was put on the adrenal glands and the rest of his body. He would have an opportunity to relax, eat nuts and berries (and a little saber-toothed tiger steak, if he was lucky). His adrenal glands would have a chance to recover.

Many people in modern society do not have the luxury of a recovery period for their overworked adrenal glands. The changes caused by the overproduction of adrenal hormones stay with them. Also, in a crowded society we get an alarm reaction over relatively minor incidents like traffic and social situations. The stimulation of the adrenal glands causes a decrease in the immune system function, so an individual under constant stress will tend to catch colds and have other immune system problems, including allergies. Blood flow to the digestive tract is decreased. Stress causes many digestive problems such as indigestion, colitis and irritable bowel. Adrenal hormones cause an increase in the blood's clotting ability, so prolonged stress can lead to arterial plaque and heart disease.

Worrying makes your adrenal glands work. Relaxing and thinking peaceful thoughts enables them to rest and heal. That is why yoga and meditation are so good for you. You go a long way in preserving your health and energy if you do not fret about things over which you have no control. It's the amount of worry and not necessarily the size of the problem that stresses your adrenal glands.

If you're sleeping late at night and you hear a noise in the house it can affect your adrenal glands. If you think it's just the wind and go back to sleep, there isn't much of an effect. If you think that someone is breaking in, you get a very strong adrenal response. You will have trouble getting back to sleep, even if you investigate and find out that the noise was indeed the wind. The stress comes from how you interpret the event, not the event itself.

If you worry a lot about little problems, you do as much damage to your adrenal glands as someone who really has a lot of stress. If you can control your worrying when under stress, you minimize the damage stress does to your health. A wise man once said that worry is interest paid in advance on money you haven't even borrowed yet.

Selye described the progression of stress on the adrenal glands as the general adaptation syndrome. The first stage is called the alarm reaction. This is when someone (with healthy adrenal glands) can perform amazingly well when the need arises. The primitive man, seeing the saber-toothed tiger, was able to run faster than he ever dreamed possible during the alarm reaction. If the stress continues, the body moves into the resistance stage, during which the adrenals become enlarged. The individual is responding to the stress and handling it. He or she may feel keyed up. The person may have cold, clammy hands, rapid pulse or reduced appetite, but hasn't begun to feel any of the more serious symptoms of the next stage, During the exhaustion stage the adrenals begin to fail to meet the demands placed upon them. During this stage, the individual begins to have a variety of symptoms including fatigue, digestive problems, obesity, depression, dizziness, fainting, allergies and many other problems. Women may respond to stress differently, but women do seem to develop problems with their adrenal glands. Excess sugar consumption can stress the adrenal glands, and many people, including women tend to eat sugar when they are stressed.

Traditional Western medicine does not recognize functional problems with the adrenal gland, unless Addison's disease (adrenal failure) is present. This is pretty amazing since medicine recognizes that the thyroid can function at various levels, including borderline hypothryoid. Traditional Western medicine has taken the view that the adrenals are either working, or they are not.

Many physicians who deal in natural health care recognize hypoadrenia and hyperadrenia. One thing these doctors look for in a patient with this problem is postural hypotension. This is when the patient's blood pressure drops when he or she stands up from a reclining position. This is interesting, because researchers recently found that patients suffering from chronic fatigue syndrome would experience a drop in blood pressure when being raised from a supine position on a tilt table. Physicians using natural health care have known about this for years. They call it the Ragland test and have been using it to tell if there is a problem with the adrenal gland.

Frequently the patient with postural hypotension feels dizzy when getting up suddenly. There are other causes for such dizziness, such as blood pressure medication, hypoglycemia and central nervous system problems. Don't diagnose yourself. Get a physical examination.

Another thing the physician may look for is a rebound pupil. Normally when a light is shined into the eye, the pupil tightly constricts. In a person with adrenal problems, the pupil will constrict and dilate again, sometimes oscillating. This is why strong light frequently bothers such a patient.

People with weak adrenal glands frequently crave coffee and sugar, as well as salt. Sugar and caffeine stimulate the adrenal glands. It's as if your adrenal glands are two horses towing a wagon load of bricks up a mountain. Sugar or caffeine is the whip you use to get the horses to keep trying. What they need to get to the top of the mountain is nourishment and a rest period.

In order to effectively treat the adrenal glands, you must eliminate as much stress from your life as possible. Emotional stress is the kind of stress most people think of when stress is mentioned, but there are many different kinds of stress. There is thermal stress from being exposed to extremes of temperature. There is physical stress, from heavy physical work, poor posture, structural misalignments, lack of sleep and being overweight. There is chemical stress from ingesting food additives, exposure to pollutants and consumption of sugar and alcohol. Changes in blood sugar are also a form of chemical stress. Skipping meals stresses the adrenal glands. Eating frequent, small meals is often very helpful, since people with adrenal problems are often hypoglycemic.

Situations are not always controllable, but stress is. Stress is cumulative. Emotional stress, structural stress and chemical stress all affect the body the same way. Your adrenal glands do not know the difference between an IRS audit, treading water or excessive sugar consumption, and excess sugar consumption will add to the stress of the IRS audit.

If you reduce the stress that you can control, stressful situations will not have as much of a physical effect on you. For instance, eating frequent meals and avoiding sugar will reduce stress on the adrenal glands. Changing how you think of stressful situations will also help preserve your health. So even if you can't do anything about Aunt Millie and Uncle Edgar coming to spend the summer, you can reduce your stress by controlling your diet. Also, how you think of the stress will make a difference in the health of your adrenal glands. Aunt Millie's handy tips on how you should raise your kids or clean your house, or Uncle Edgar's penchant for eating everything that isn't nailed down (without offering to pay for groceries) won't make you crazy if you don't focus on it.

If there is a situation in your life that you can't control, reduce the stress in the areas of your life that you can control. Also, try to focus on the positive areas of your life and not the one or two things that really stress you out. If your job or your relationship situation is not exactly perfect, or not completely under your control, you can still reduce the effect stress has on your body and adrenal glands by reducing other forms of stress that you can control and by controlling what you focus your mind on.

If you can't change your work situation, then improve your diet and get plenty of rest. Change how you think about your job situation. Focus on the positive: You have a job, and you are able to eat regular meals. (Much of the world doesn't.) Just do the best you can and think of the things you can't control in positive terms. Jesus says in Luke 12:25, "And which of you with taking thought can add to his stature one cubit?" Or, to quote my teacher and spiritual advisor, Yogi Babaganoush, "Chill out man." Think to yourself, "What could be good about this situation?" Then take a minute to really look for positive answers.

Hanging on to anxiety over past situations is stressful. Thought has power. Worry gives you all of the physiologic responses of Selye's rats or the caveman facing the saber-toothed tiger. It's a waste of energy and it undermines your health. This is one reason so many religions stress forgiveness. Forgiveness doesn't let the person who offended you off of the hook—it lets you off of the hook.

Your adrenal glands simply don't know the difference between imagined danger and real danger. This is why meditation and biofeedback have been so valuable in controlling stress. Doctors are beginning to find that laughter helps the prognosis of cancer patients. They even have patients watch sitcoms in the hospital: "Mr. Smith, it's time for your chemotherapy and *'I Love Lucy'* reruns."

Minimizing chemical stress is also important. We have plenty of chemical stress today. Environmental pollution, food additives, sugar, alcohol and caffeine contribute stress to your adrenal glands. You must remove chemical stresses from your diet—effortlessly and without putting yourself under pressure. Gradually improve your diet by removing chemical additives. Move toward a more organic way of eating. Enjoy the change without fretting over how your diet isn't perfect yet.

Ironically, stress often makes you crave the foods that are bad for you. While under stress, it's hard to be diligent in keeping additives out of the diet. Patients often complain that they have no time and can't eat properly. Lack of time really isn't the problem because raw nuts, fruits and vegetables do not have to be cooked and take no time to prepare. If it was sex, and not food preparation, you'd find the time. Lack of time is usually used as an excuse to give in to craving the wrong foods. Once you understand that, you can eat healthily with little effort.

Eating sugar and skipping meals are two things that are especially stressful to the adrenal glands. Your adrenals work to keep your blood sugar level. Eating sugar causes a temporary increase in blood sugar, which soon drops. Skipping meals also causes the blood sugar to drop. The adrenals then have to work to increase the blood sugar. Hypoadrenia and hypoglycemia (low blood sugar) usually exist together.

There are other things you can do to treat the adrenal glands. In many natural health techniques there are several reflex points that will improve adrenal function when manually stimulated. Chiropractic adjustments, massage and other types of bodywork reduce stress. Vitamin supplements, such as vitamin C, vitamin B complex and other nutrients are often helpful.

One form of treatment, which is rather controversial, is the use of glandular supplements. Many practitioners frequently give their patients a supplement made from the adrenal glands of a cow or a sheep (with the active hormone removed). Biotics Research uses neonatal bovine adrenal tissue to make its adrenal supplement (Cytozyme-AD). The neonatal source is a purer source than glandular tissue taken from adult animals. There is some evidence to support the value of these supplements. Radioactively labeled adrenal glandular substance has been found to go to the adrenal glands of the individual injected with adrenal substance. Biotics makes another adrenal supplement, ADHS, which has no glandular tissue.

A few years ago when doctors working with nutrition and natural health began to address problems with the adrenal glands, they called the problem functional hypoadrenia. Now that we can test adrenal hormone levels with salivary testing, we realize that hyperadrenia is often the problem. When the rats began to tread water, the adrenal glands hypertrophied and increased their production of hormones. This is actually the beginning of health problems. Sugar and salt cravings, back and knee pain, fatigue, hypoglycemia, poor immune function and many of the other problems we used to associate with hypoadrenia actually happen when there is too much adrenal output.

You may have heard about DHEA and of the findings that observe that DHEA levels drop as we age. This has prompted an increase in the sale of DHEA as an anti-aging substance. Self-medicating with DHEA is not a good idea. DHEA comes from the same chemical that makes cortisol (an adrenal hormone). Stress causes the body to make cortisol instead of DHEA, so cortisol levels increase and DHEA levels decrease. One of the things ADHS (Biotics' nonglandular adrenal supplement) does is to correct this imbalance. In general, ADHS is given to support hyperadrenia and Cytozyme-AD is given to support hypoadrenia.

One of the problems with some brands of glandular supplement is inconsistency in the potency and the quality of the products. It may even be possible, that in some brands, not all of the hormones are removed. If the hormone is not completely removed from the gland, it works like a drug and can create problems. This is one reason that you should seek the help of a health care provider trained in nutrition. He or she can help to make sure that the supplements you take are not only appropriate, but of acceptable quality. Also, other supplements like vitamins B complex and C, minerals and essential fatty acids can help to support the adrenal gland.

Clinically, when a glandular substance is given to the patient who needs it, the results are often dramatic. Frequently patients suffering from adrenal insufficiency improve when they take an adrenal glandular. They sometimes improve when given a glandular made of thymus. Frequently the thymus improves the immune system of someone suffering from allergies.

The intention here is not to get everyone to run out and take glandular substances. In fact, they can be harmful in some patients. This is only to inform you of some of the treatments available and that this is a subject that warrants further investigation. It would be interesting to see more research done on glandular substances. If this is something that you think you may want to try, get help from a physician who understands it. The issue of supplement quality alone makes it necessary to get professional expertise.

Some herbs, like ephedra or mah wong stimulate the adrenals. Be careful with products like this; the herb stimulates the adrenals, it doesn't heal them or strengthen them. You initially feel great, but the herb is a stress to the adrenals. Ephedra is in a lot of weight loss formulas. Once again, don't treat yourself. You may end up like the unfortunate Mr. Needlebrain.

You can improve your adrenal function without stressing the glands. The following steps will improve your health and help you to overcome the effects of stress:

- **Meditation:** Meditation, yoga, Tai Chi or simple deep breathing exercises can help you bring stress under control. Much of the damage that stress does to your health is not due to any external factors, but rather how your mind interprets those factors. Meditation and other techniques help to reduce the harm of stress by quieting the mind.
- **Sports and hobbies:** Meditation and yoga may be a little "New Age" for some people. Hobbies are a good solution for these people. Most hobbies are relaxing; your mind has to focus on a simple task rather than on sources of stress.
- **Exercise:** Moderate aerobic exercise is good. This is exercise that uses large muscles repetitively and is mild enough that you can carry on a normal conversation during the activity. Anaerobic exercise (working so hard that you can't carry on a normal conversation) can be stressful and should be limited while the adrenal glands are recovering.
- **Diet:** There are many types of stress. Chemical, physical, thermal and mental stresses can all cause harm to the body. Stress is cumulative. A stressful job situation is compounded by a poor diet. Eat small, frequent meals, avoid chemical additives and sugar, refined carbohydrates and hydrogenated oil. Eat plenty of vegetables and make sure that you get enough protein. At mealtime relax and focus on enjoying your food, don't eat on the run. Snack frequently and keep your blood sugar from dropping.
- **Supplementation:** We have already discussed glandulars and ADHS. Stress also depletes vitamins B and C. Stress causes you to excrete

minerals (especially calcium and magnesium) into your urine. Your health care provider can help you with additional supplementation.

## Structural Stress

Poor posture, bad ergonomics and tight muscles can be stressful and drain your energy. A muscle that is in spasm uses the same amount of energy as a muscle doing work. Your body doesn't know the difference between physical work and having a muscle spasm. Those tight upper back muscles at the end of a day's work are the equivalent of lifting something over and over again; the muscle uses energy and produces waste. It's doing work, but it's not accomplishing anything but making you tired and uncomfortable. It can be a major cause of fatigue.

Poor posture can affect your breathing, muscle tone and ultimately your energy level. Holding your head forward makes the muscles in your upper back and neck work very hard. It can cause muscle spasm. Poor posture also causes you to breathe shallowly, reducing the amount of oxygen reaching the tissues and reducing the flow of the lymphatic system.

Good posture when viewed from the front consists of having you head balanced over your pelvis, hips level, shoulders level and head level. If you look at your body from the side, the ears should be directly above the shoulders and hip joints. The ear, shoulder and hip joint should form a line that is perpendicular to the ground. The spine should be straight, allowing only for the normal curves of the spine (which are the lumbar and cervical lordosis and the thoracic kyphosis).

Ergonomics literally means "laws of work" in Latin. It is the rules for posture, designing workstations, lifting and using proper body mechanics. In a job that is sedentary, involves staying in one position for a long time, or has repetitive motion, it is best to minimize the stress on the body. That is the purpose of ergonomics.

If you sit, the chair should support your lumbar spine, and should have arm rests. The height of the chair should be adjustable to enable your thighs to be level and your feet to be level and on the ground.. Also, the chair should have wheels on it so you can get to other areas of your workstation without reaching. You should not have to reach higher than your shoulders or lower than your hips. If something is above your shoulders, use a step stool to reach it. Things that you use frequently should be within easy reach and you should not spend the day bending down or reaching up.

Working on a computer presents some unique ergonomic problems. Using proper ergonomics will help to make sure that you don't come down with "floppy disk" or other structural problems. Carpal tunnel syndrome is common in people who work on computers all day. Resting your wrists on a foam pad that sits at the base of your keyboard will help prevent carpal tunnel.

Carpal tunnel can be treated by correcting the alignment of the wrist bones. Another idea is that many "carpal tunnel" sufferers are actually suffering from a kind of compartment syndrome. This means that the muscles of the forearm swell a little with repetitive use and the swelling creates some of the nerve pressure. There is one method that is sometimes effective for relieving wrist, arm or hand pain caused by repetitive use. Massage the forearm with ice until it gets a little numb. (You can freeze water in a small paper cup and use it as an applicator.) Then rub your arm hard in straight lines from the elbow to the wrist, using your thumb. Do this all around the arm. This is called fascial flushing. It loosens the fascia around the muscles of the forearm, relieving some of the pressure. Supplementation with $B_{12}$, folic acid, magnesium and essential fatty acids often helps. Vitamin $B_6$ has also

97

been recommended for patients with carpal tunnel, and does provide relief for some.

People working with computers tend to hold their head motionless for long periods of time. This is hard on your neck and upper back. Make absolutely sure that the screen is at eye level and that you don't hold your head forward, or look up or down for long periods of time. When working on a computer, do not go more than 10 minutes without moving your neck and shoulders. Set a timer, and every 10 minutes stretch and rotate your neck. This will reduce fatigue and spasm in the neck and upper back. If muscles fatigue easily, then you may need essential fatty acids and supplementation with flax or fish oil may be beneficial. Also, people who are deficient in essential fatty acids should strictly avoid deep-fried foods, hydrogenated and partially hydrogenated oils.

It is helpful if your monitor is capable of moving. Changing the monitor position throughout the day will help to reduce the strain on your neck and upper back.

Laptop computers are very bad ergonomically. The monitor is low and the keyboard is small. Using one forces your head forward and down and you shoulders rounded. If you use a laptop, use a separate monitor and keyboard whenever possible.

One of the absolutely worst things you can do while working on a computer is to sit for long periods of time, motionless, with your head turned. People doing word processing and copying documents frequently sit this way. It is a common source of neck pain.

People who make their living talking on the telephone often suffer from neck pain and spasm. Many are in the habit of holding the receiver between their ear and shoulder. That is just asking for pain and muscle spasm. Use a headset if you spend a lot of time on the telephone.

Try this exercise: Let your head (but only your head) hang as far forward as is comfortable. With your fingertips, press firmly just below the base of the skull. Use a comfortable pressure to make tiny circles from the center out to your ears and back again.

Exercises to strengthen the muscles of your neck and those between your shoulder blades are also helpful. Sitting up straight and pinching your shoulder blades together will strengthen the muscles that hold your shoulders back. Hold it for 15 seconds. Neck retractions are also good for people who sit at a computer a lot, or who have chronic neck tightness. Extend your neck by moving your head backward. Keep your head perfectly level while doing this. Hold your head in this position for 15 seconds. Do 5–10 repetitions of each exercise each day.

If you stand and work at a counter, it should be at a proper height so that you can work without bending. If you stand for long periods of time, it helps to put your foot on a small footrest about six inches in height. Change which foot is on the footrest from time to time.

Lifting should be done without bending at the waist. Bend your knees to get close to what you are lifting. Keep your back straight and bring the item in as close to your body as you can get it. Lift even small objects properly. The combination of bending at the waist and twisting the spine is very stressful and can cause you to injure your low back.

Even lifting something small off of the floor will cause a severe back injury if the person bends at the waist and twists to one side while bending. How often have you heard someone say, "I just picked up my pen (or the cap off the toothpaste, a nickel or my false teeth), and I got the worst pain in my back?"

Ninety-eight percent of all Americans will have back pain at some point in their lives. There are specific back exercises that will help prevent back injury. If you are a sedentary individual, light exercise will generally help your posture, breathing and muscle tone. Structural stress can be handled in several ways. Stretching, exercise, good posture and proper ergonomics will help prevent the fatigue caused by poor body mechanics. Often it is necessary to get outside help with your structural problems. Chiropractic, massage, Rolfing, and other types of bodywork will help you to feel better.

## Muscle Tension and Subluxation

Poor posture creates tension in the small muscles in the spine, called multifidi. These muscles are an inch or two long and connect individual vertebrae. Chronically poor posture creates spasms in these muscles, which in turn cause distortions in the alignment of individual vertebra. These misalignments are called subluxations. They can be caused by old injuries, poor body mechanics and even chemical stress.

Have you have ever had a cast on your arm, leg or other broken bone, and that cast kept a joint from moving? Remember how hard it was to move the joint when the cast was removed? The spine is dozens of joints and is meant to be highly mobile. Chronic subluxations and fixations create stiffness and lack of mobility similar to that of a joint that has been placed in a cast.

Virtually every nerve in the body passes through the spine. When the spine contains subluxations, fixations and muscle spasm, the nervous system is affected. The obvious manifestation of this is pain and discomfort, which are caused by stimulation (or irritation) of the nerves that emerge from the spine.

Sometimes the pain is severe; sometimes it is merely annoying. Pain is what brings most people to chiropractors. Chiropractors adjust (manipulate) subluxations and fixations to relieve pain and discomfort. It works very well. Chiropractic, as we know it, has been around for a hundred years. Spinal manipulation, however, has been practiced since the time of the ancient Egyptians and has a pretty good track record of improving health and relieving pain.

Chiropractic has been pigeonholed into treating pain. This has more to do with the depth in which the insurance companies can understand chiropractic and the chiropractors' desire to become mainstream health providers than reality. Chiropractic adjustments affect the autonomic and central nervous systems. Originally chiropractic was used to get the nervous system to heal the body—not simple pain relief. Early chiropractors would probably not recognize the profession as it is.

The spinal nerves are responsible for feeling pain (and other sensations) and for the movement of muscles. They emerge from the spinal column and are responsible for feeling and movement throughout the body. Pain, weakness and other symptoms caused by irritation of spinal nerves are what usually bring people to chiropractors. To most people, the value of chiropractic is its ability to relieve neck, back and other musculoskeletal pain. Even chronic distortions of the spine, while taking a little more time, can be relieved through chiropractic care.

## Chiropractic and the Nervous System

While it is clear to many people that chiropractic is effective in treating neck, back and musculoskeletal pain, they may not fully realize that chiropractic helps the function of other parts of the nervous system, the autonomic nervous system and the central nervous system. In the autonomic nervous system there are clusters of nerves, called ganglia alongside of the spine. The ganglia handle automatic functions; that is, they work autonomously. When you eat, you don't have to tell your stomach to produce acid for digestion. When you run, you don't have to tell your heart to beat faster to supply blood and oxygen to your legs. These functions happen automatically. Think of the brain as the president of the company. The president isn't involved with every detail of the running of that company. There are heads of various departments, marketing, accounting, sales etc. These department heads are like the ganglia of the autonomic nervous system.

Actually the above explanation is way too simplistic, but this isn't a neurology text. For example, chiropractors have been successfully treating bed wetting in children for years. It doesn't work for every single child, but it works for enough children to make it worth a try. Some chiropractors have explained this by saying that they are affecting the nerve that goes from the spine to the bladder. Actually, an area in the front of the brain is responsible for overriding the urge to urinate. In all likelihood the chiropractors are improving the function of the neurological pathways from that area of the brain. Indeed, proprioceptive input (a fancy name for joint stimulation) facilitates many neurological pathways.

People often think of chiropractors as treating bones, but in reality they treat the nervous system. If you take a rubber band and put it around your arm, your hand will become numb, tingle and then ache. You have interfered with the nerve and blood supply. Similarly, subluxations and fixations affect your body. Spinal nerves are affected, causing pain and weakness and the autonomic nervous system is affected causing dysfunction in various organs.

When you place a rubber band around your arm, the effects are felt in a few minutes. Pressure from subluxations and fixations, when chronic, are usually subtle and their effects are felt over time.

Relieving subluxations and fixations creates a sense of well-being and improves health. Ask any person who has been going to a chiropractor how they feel after an adjustment. Chiropractic is effective for relieving pain, but its real strength lies in its ability to improve the health of the nervous system and the rest of the body. *Chiropractic is a holistic profession that helps to ensure a lifetime of good health.*

Chiropractic is a great way to improve your structural well-being. Frequently patients will notice that they feel much better after going to the chiropractor. Patients often report a sense of lightness and well-being that goes beyond the correction of the specific ache or pain that brought them to the chiropractor in the first place.

Most people have structural problems, slight distortions in the spine, slight muscle imbalances and tightness that are not painful. The imbalances create a kind of epicritical pain, which the patient is probably not consciously aware of. It's like a loud fan; after a while you don't notice it. When the fan is turned off, you say to yourself, "Wow, that sounds better." A chiropractic adjustment removes these slight distortions. The patient feels better, even if he or she didn't have a specific pain.

The following exercise will illustrate the importance of structural balance and how posture affects your mental attitude. Stand and breathe as if you are depressed; slump your shoulders, hang your head down and breathe shallowly. Notice how you feel. If you do the exercise, you really begin to feel depressed. Now, stand up straight, shoulder back and head held high; breathe deeply and put a silly grin on your face. You do it and begin to feel really happy and energetic.

How you carry yourself affects your mood. There is a connection between structural balance and psychological well-being. The way you carry your body affects your mood and your energy level. Chiropractors and other body workers have known this for years. To put yourself in a good mood and increase your energy, use your posture, breathing, facial expressions and body language. Simply stand straight, breathe deeply, look up and put a grin on your face. You can use your mental focus to improve the feeling. Remember a time when you felt wonderful (confident, energetic, happy—whatever emotion you wish). Mentally take yourself back to that time. Model, or recreate every gesture. Model your posture, facial expression and mental feelings. Since your mind doesn't know the difference between something real or something imagined, you really do begin to feel the energy and confidence you had in the past. It's amazing; you can change your mood and energy level in an instant.

## Exercise

There are benefits to exercise other than the ones that are commonly discussed by fitness experts. Increased strength, endurance and cardiovascular fitness are only the beginning. Exercise also reduces structural stress by strengthening muscles and improving posture.

Exercise actually increases serotonin production effectively and without the side effects of anti-depressant drugs. One of the best treatments for depression is to simply get the body moving.

Exercise improves tissue oxygenation. During exercise you breathe deeply and your heart rate increases, which increases the amount of oxygen the cells receive. Deep breathing and muscle movement during exercise also increase lymphatic circulation, improving the cells' ability to eliminate waste.

You may be so tired that a nap is a lot more appealing to you than any kind of physical activity. If you are normally sedentary, exercise will actually increase your energy. Stand up right now, and take a few deep breaths. Now, run in place for 30 seconds.

You'll notice, after doing the exercise, that you have more energy than you had two paragraphs ago. Being sedentary is fatiguing. Shallow breathing and lack of muscle motion in the sedentary individual lead to poor lymphatic circulation, poor oxygenation and fatigue. Sedentary people sit there stewing in their own wastes, tired, but not ready for sleep. They may want some stimulation, but don't have the energy to do anything. What are the most likely forms of stimulus such an individual would choose? Food and television, of course. They provide diversion, without requiring any effort.

Of course, using food and TV for diversion can make you have the dimensions of a marine mammal and be tired all of the time. You may have even created a little canyon on your end of the couch or may have an easy chair with the springs partially broken down. There is nothing quite as comfortable as a couch or chair that is contour-shaped to your rear end. The modern age is truly wonderful; you can perform less activity than a dead person and still be entertained.

A few years ago I gained 45 pounds by becoming devoted to carry-out food and bad television. My wife was pregnant, and, as a sensitive husband, I was determined to gain weight with her, pound for pound. It's easy to gain weight and feel exhausted. TV and junk food really do the job.

If you are not very active, exercise may be unthinkable. It was for me; until my landlord insisted that I lose weight or move to the first floor. He was afraid for the safety of the tenants living below me. It's a good thing we were in Chicago, because it was possible to bribe the building inspectors and keep them from condemning the building from the structural stress caused by my weight gain.

I began jogging until the department of streets and sanitation complained and threatened to have me pay for the increased repair needed to the streets and sidewalks in my neighborhood. One of the potholes I created attracted spelunkers from all over Illinois. The Illinois National Guard used it to practice rappelling. The city finally repaired the pothole after someone was injured while hang gliding across it. It made me sad to see it repaired because I had been making a nice living by selling donkey rides to the bottom.

I switched to a stationary bicycle, which worked pretty well once we'd reinforced the seat and frame. It was surprising how much better I felt once I began exercising. I was still big enough to influence the tides when I walked near Lake Michigan, but I had a lot more energy.

Your exercise program will depend a lot on what kind of shape you are in and what your goals are. First of all, you should discuss this topic with your health care provider. If you have not exercised in a while or if you are overweight, you need to start easy.

A book worth getting is *In Fitness and in Health* by Dr. Phil Maffetone. He does a very good job at distinguishing aerobic exercise and anaerobic exercise and knowing which type of exercise you need. Think of a pyramid: Aerobic exercise is like the base. Aerobic exercise is easy movement of large muscle groups. If you are doing aerobic exercise, you can converse easily without being out of breath. Your heart rate is around 180 minus your age. This is to be distinguished from "aerobics" that people do in health clubs or with videotapes. These exercise programs usually include some anaerobic activity. Aerobic exercise means that the heart rate does not go higher than 180 minus your age and you do not get out of breath. If you get out of breath, you are doing anaerobic exercise.

Anaerobic exercise is analogous to the height of the pyramid. It is what increases your performance and helps you attain many of the goals of exercise like strength, speed and weight loss. You are doing anaerobic exercise when you are out of breath or can't talk normally while exercising.

If you are just doing aerobic exercise you won't progress much. Your weight loss will plateau and your strength and endurance will not increase. You see this a lot in people who are trying to lose weight. They do the same exercise like a treadmill or a stationary bicycle without pushing themselves much. They lose weight for a while and then just stop. Usually anaerobic activity will help these people to achieve their goals.

Some people overdo it with anaerobic activity. People who intensely train for sports, like marathon runners, tend to do too much anaerobic activity. People who push themselves to gain performance also seem to have more injuries. Too much anaerobic activity is a stress to the adrenal glands and can predispose the exerciser to injury or chronic pain. These are the runners with chronic knee pain, weight lifters with tendonitis, quarterbacks with chronic shoulder problems and so on. If you use the pyramid analogy, it's like having a very tall structure with a little tiny base. It isn't very stable.

People who want to train for performance will do well to pay attention to nutrition. Not eating hydrogenated oils and supplementing with essential fatty acids is a good start. Strictly avoiding refined sugar and refined white flour is also very important.

Get the help of a professional to help you with supplementation—some of the advice going around gyms is questionable.

Another thing that is very important during exercise is to properly warm up, for at least 10 minutes at the beginning and to properly cool down at the end. The warm up increases blood flow to the muscles and increases flexibility. At the end of the exercise, cool down for at least 10 minutes, it helps to re-establish normal circulation and prevents blood from pooling in the muscles.

You need a balance of both aerobic and anaerobic exercise. If you are out of shape or new to an exercise regimen, you need to build an aerobic base. Spend a month or two just going on a treadmill or stationary bicycle. Later you can add weight lifting or more intense cardiovascular activity.

Dr. Maffetone shows you how to know how to balance aerobic and anaerobic activity in his book. The book shows you how to test yourself using a heart rate monitor while you exercise. It can give you more detailed information about exercise than is presented here.

Your pulse can be taken at your radial or your carotid arteries. The bone of the forearm that is on the same side as the thumb is called the radius. The radial pulse is found just inside (medial to) the radius, near where the wrist bends. The carotid pulse is found on either side of your windpipe. The carotid pulse is a little stronger and will be easier to find than the radial pulse. Or, if you don't mind spending a few dollars, you can buy a heart monitor.

If you still can't find your pulse, jump up and down a few times and try again. Now just count the number of beats for one minute. If you are lazy like I am, count the beats for 15 seconds and multiply by 4. If you are really out of shape, you may be surprised at how little activity it takes to get your heart rate up.

## Sleep

I was sitting in my living room at 3:00 A.M. with my suddenly social six-month-old daughter, and two things occurred to me. First, until then, I'd managed to avoid talking about one of the most obvious causes of fatigue, which is not getting enough sleep. Secondly, we were once offered a lot of money for this lively infant by a band of infertile yuppies.

Obviously, if you are going to have enough energy, you should get enough sleep. You may have other reasons, such as job obligations, a too active social life or a nocturnal neighbor who likes to play the saxophone (some folks in Harlem have reported having this problem), for not getting enough sleep. If lack of sleep is a problem for you, the best suggestion is to try to get more.

For many, getting to sleep and staying asleep is a problem. If it is, please come over and watch my daughter. Actually, there are some things that you can do to help yourself to sleep. For years many people took tryptophan. That was before the FDA banned it because some people became sick from a bad batch. Tryptophan is a precursor for serotonin and melotonin; 5-hydroxy tryptophan is still available and it too is a precursor to serotonin and melotonin.

People under stress, with overactive adrenal glands have trouble sleeping. Biotics Research makes a product called De-Stress that works very well for some people, especially if there is an adrenal component to their sleep problem. It is made from a protein found in milk. French researchers found that this protein can favorably affect sleep patterns. It can also calm the adrenal glands. When De-Stress works, it works well. It doesn't work for everyone, but some of the patients who take it simply stop having problems sleeping. Some patients continue to sleep well after discontinuing

De-*Stress*. De-*Stress* is also a useful supplement for people who are keyed up and have trouble calming down.

There is some evidence that magnesium supplementation will help some people get to sleep. Calcium works for some patients. Chewing five or six calcium/magnesium tablets right before going to sleep will often help you fall asleep.

Low blood sugar often causes an individual to wake up and have trouble getting back to sleep. Many times eating a piece of fruit and going back to bed works. If you wake up after a few hours of sleep and have trouble going back to sleep you should stop eating refined sugar and refined carbohydrates. Snack frequently and make sure that you are eating enough protein. Patients with this problem are often deficient in B vitamins, especially thiamin. Often they have low blood pressure and fatigue. Biotics Research makes Bio 3B-G, a B complex with a little extra thiamin. It is a low-dose product. If you chew a tablet several times throughout the day, it will often help resolve this problem.

Different nutrient deficiencies can be at the root of insomnia. Folic acid and magnesium both are important cofactors for producing serotonin and melotonin, contributing neurotransmitters that help you to calm down and get to sleep.

Avoiding protein late at night helps some people to sleep. Protein contains tyrosine, an amino acid that can act as a stimulant to the nervous system. Eating a meal that is mostly carbohydrate late in the day will increase serotonin levels in the brain. Serotonin acts as a sedative. You don't want to go to bed too hungry or after having eaten too much.

Problems with the digestive system can contribute to sleep patterns. Changing your diet for the better will help improve sleep. Supplementation with digestive enzymes or hydrochloric acid may also be helpful here.

If you have trouble getting to sleep, don't just lie there and worry about how much sleep you're not getting. Get up and do something relaxing. Read or work on a puzzle. When you become sleepy, go back to bed (and tell your internal dialog to shut up).

Other things you can do to improve your sleeping include avoiding stimulants such as caffeine and nicotine late in the day. If you can completely give them up, so much the better. Also give up alcohol. Exercise, but not too late in the day. There is evidence to suggest that people who exercise get a better quality sleep than those who do not. Exercise actually increases serotonin production. Also, don't take naps. Getting up at the same time every morning makes for better sleep patterns.

Sometimes sleep apnea is a problem. People with sleep apnea are people who snore and who stop breathing when they snore. When they stop breathing, it is very stressful on the cardiovascular system and it keeps the individual from having quality sleep. It's actually pretty dangerous. People with sleep apnea tend not to remember their dreams and feel sleepy, no matter how much sleep they get. Losing weight and getting in shape often helps. Some holistic doctors treat these patients for allergies. The medical approach involves using oxygen under slight pressure to keep the airway open. If you suspect this is a problem for you, talk to your doctor.

**OTHER HEALTH ISSUES**

Improving your diet and getting rid of bad habits like smoking and drinking alcohol will improve your health and energy. Some people need a little more help than lifestyle changes. There are people who have a much healthier lifestyle than their friends who have no symptoms, but they struggle with their health.

Let's go back to our automobile analogy. If your car doesn't start and you've checked the gas, made sure that it was in neutral, and made sure that the battery has a charge, the car still may not start. The problem may still be relatively easy to fix. You may need spark plugs, a new Bendix spring, a new solenoid or some other relatively inexpensive repair. Similarly, problems with digestion, the endocrine system, allergies or structural balance may interfere with you enjoying excellent health and energy.

## DIGESTION

If you were chronically ill and you could only choose one area of your body to treat, your best, first choice would be to treat the digestive system. Problems with digestion can be the root of fatigue, skin problems, allergies, arthritis and just about any chronic symptom that you can name.

Digesting food takes a great deal of energy. Inefficient digestion wastes energy, causes fatigue after meals and can cause malabsorption of nutrients. You could be eating a nutrient-rich diet and still not be absorbing all of the vitamins and minerals. Incomplete digestion can also cause the creation of toxic waste products that are absorbed by the body. These toxins can irritate the lining of the GI tract, and place a burden on the kidneys and liver. They can cause fatigue, much the same way that a hangover causes fatigue. A hangover is merely a toxic state.

Eating refined foods, taking drugs (prescription and otherwise), chemical additives, alcohol, environmental pollution, a diet that is deficient in fiber and nutrients, exposure to pathogenic organisms, eating too rapidly, and underproduction of hydrochloric acid and enzymes all can cause problems with digestion.

112

Even having not been breastfed as an infant can cause future digestive problems.

The GI tract is a muscular tube. Muscle fibers encircle it and muscle fibers run along it. The fibers can pinch together to move food through the tube. That movement is called peristalsis. It's like the movement you see in a cartoon when a snake swallows an animal.

The tube runs from the mouth to the anus. Food inside the tube is still technically outside of the body. Cells lining the tube act as a barrier between the digesting food and the bloodstream. They produce enzymes to chemically break down the food. These cells also selectively absorb nutrients. The tube is in several sections. Each section is defined by the type of enzyme secreted and the type of absorption that takes place. The mouth, esophagus, stomach, small intestine, large intestine and rectum are all parts of the same tube.

Thoroughly chewing your food will enable the stomach to work more efficiently. If you have a piece of iron that weighs one ounce, and you place it in a beaker of acid, it will dissolve much more slowly than an ounce of iron shavings. If you thoroughly chew your food, you will eat less, absorb more nutrient and place less stress on your digestive system than if you don't. The next part of the digestive tract, the stomach, is an out pouching of the tube. The stomach produces hydrochloric acid and the enzyme, pepsin, which work to break down protein.

After the food leaves the stomach through the pylorus it goes into the next part of the tube, the small intestine. The small intestine is about 20 feet long and about an inch in diameter. The inner surface is ridged, giving the interior an accordion shape. The lining of the small intestine is full of fingerlike projections, known as villi, which are about a millimeter long. Each individual cell on the villi has miniature projections known as microvilli. The design of the small intestine, with the increased surface area, enhances the absorption of nutrients. Of course, swallowing a battleship-sized lump of food will make absorption less efficient.

The purpose of these projections, the villi and the microvilli, is to increase the surface area of the small intestine. If the small intestine was just a flat tube, it would have a four-square-yard area. With the added surface area of the ridges, villi and microvilli, the surface of the small intestine is more than 400 square yards, larger than a tennis court.

Alcoholism, other diseases and even poor diet can lead to a situation known as villous atrophy. This is a flattening of the villi and the microvilli. The loss of surface area decreases the absorption of nutrients from the small intestine. This can happen from drug or alcohol use, infection or allergic reactions. In some patients, an allergy to wheat and other grains can cause irritation to the lining of the small intestine and villous atrophy. As much as half of the surface area of the small intestine can be lost, causing digestive disturbance, nutrient deficiencies and, of course, fatigue. Folic acid is one nutrient that is very important for keeping the villi intact and healthy.

The first part of the small intestine is called the *duodenum*, which is Latin for 12. It is about 12 inches long (hence the name). This is where the pancreas adds its digestive enzymes and liver adds bile. Protease, lipase and amylase are from the pancreas. These enzymes digest protein, fat and starch respectively. Bile from the liver helps to digest fat.

The small intestine is about 20 feet long. Most of the nutrients from the meal are absorbed in the small intestine. There are three sections to the small intestine, the duodenum, just mentioned; the jejunum; and the ileum. The small intestine changes morphology over the course of its 20 feet. In the upper small intestine the villi are packed close together, and there is more surface area than in the lower small intestine. Most of the absorption of nutrients occurs in the small intestine. Carbohydrates, fats and proteins are broken down and absorbed there, as well as vitamins and minerals.

The ileocecal valve separates the large and the small intestine. It prevents the backflow of fecal contents into the small intestines. Its function is a lot like keeping your septic tank from flowing into your well water.

Although the practice is not generally recognized by medicine, certain natural health care practitioners work on the ileocecal valve, either opening or closing it. These practitioners believe that the valve can be stuck in the open position, allowing fecal backwash into the small intestine, creating toxicity symptoms. It can also be stuck in the closed position, allowing the digested food to ferment in the small intestine, also creating toxicity. The techniques do seem to help alleviate toxicity symptoms such as headache, muscle soreness and fatigue.

The large intestine is only about five feet long, but it is much larger in diameter than the small intestine. The large intestine absorbs electrolytes and water. About half of the volume of stool consists of microorganisms. Bacteria in the large intestine produce vitamin K, which is important to blood coagulation, and vitamin $B_{12}$.

Since everything you consume has to pass through the digestive tract, problems with it can cause other chronic or systemic problems. Good digestion is necessary to good health.

Food begins its journey through the digestive tract in the mouth. Chewing is the first phase of digestion. The food is ground into small pieces and mixed with saliva, which lubricates the food. Saliva contains the enzyme, amylase, which digests carbohydrates. Chewing food thoroughly is vital to good digestion. If the food is not broken down by chewing and mixed with saliva, it will not be easy to digest.

Eating in a hurry creates problems with digestion. Let's say that you have the bologna sandwich we talked about in the food additive section, and you're in a hurry. It's a nice soft food, easy to swallow. A couple of bites and you can get it down your throat before the mustard hits your lap, letting out the occasional snort to let some air in.

The next part of the digestive tract is the esophagus. It has no enzymes, and does nothing to digest food, except to move it to the stomach. You can, however, have problems with your esophagus. Wolfing down that bologna sandwich can be the cause of some of those problems.

The esophagus has a muscular valve that separates it from the contents of the stomach. The diaphragm also helps keep the esophagus separate from the stomach. The diaphragm is the muscle that spreads across the bottom of the chest cavity and enables you to breathe. It keeps the chest and abdominal cavities separate. The esophagus travels through the chest cavity and passes through an opening in the diaphragm called the curia. It is meant to be tight around the bottom of the esophagus, keeping the stomach and esophagus separate. The separation of the esophagus from the stomach is important since the stomach contains extremely strong acid and the lining of the esophagus is not resistant to acid.

Swallowing a bowling-ball-sized lump of white bread and bologna hurtles it down the esophagus toward the stomach like a boulder heading for the coyote in a "Roadrunner" cartoon. (Maybe it was Acme Bologna.) It hits the opening and squeezes through the crura, like John Madden trying to get into tight Lycra stretch pants.

Eating rapidly and swallowing large chunks of food can cause the crura and the muscular valve to stop being an effective barrier between the stomach and esophagus. This causes gastric reflux, or acid in the esophagus. It causes burning and discomfort. The cells lining the esophagus are not resistant to the acid in the stomach.

A hiatal hernia can also develop. This is a situation where the top part of the stomach is actually above the diaphragm, allowing stomach acid to enter the esophagus. It can cause burning and pain and can even mimic a heart attack.

Acid from the stomach is irritating to the esophagus, causing a burning sensation. The burning seems to be caused by too much acid. After all, the TV has been telling you about acid indigestion for years, so you take an antacid. The ad says, "If you eat too well, demand Di-Gel." It should say, "If you eat like an idiot, demand Di-Gel." Or, how do you spell relief? "CHEW-YOUR-FOOD" or "USE-SOME-SENSE."

**Hydrochloric Acid, Reflux and Nutrient Absorption**

Hypochlorhydra is a state where the stomach produces less hydrochloric acid than normal. Achlorhydra is the complete absence of stomach acid. Both conditions are recognized by medicine and described in standard physiology texts; however, the medical view is that even in the absence of stomach acid, the pancreas produces enough enzymes so that digestion is nearly normal.

Most efforts by doctors to help digestion are to give substances to neutralize stomach acid. There are many antacids available over the counter. Doctors have commonly prescribed antacids in the past to patients suffering from ulcers, although it is now known that ulcers are often caused by a bacterium and are usually treated with a course of antibiotics.

Hypochlorhydra is one of those things that is treated by doctors dealing in natural health care, but is not considered to be a problem by doctors who deal in sickness care. In this discussion, what follows is the view held by some doctors who are involved in natural health care. Just realize that not every doctor is going to agree with what is written here.

Physicians dealing in natural health care view hypochlorhydra as a problem that leads to malabsorption of minerals, poor protein digestion, vitamin $B_{12}$ deficiency and even problems with bowel flora. The problems caused by hypochlorhydra can lead to a number of subclinical complaints including gas, bloating, fatigue and even depression.

Hypochlorhydra creates deficiencies in a number of nutrients. Your body needs acid in order to absorb iron, calcium and several other minerals Vitamin $B_{12}$ and essential amino acids are common deficiencies that accompany hypochlorhydra. Taking antacids can make these deficiencies worse.

People who do not produce enough stomach acid tend to dislike meat. Many vegetarians say that they feel better if they do not eat meat. A meal containing meat may cause them to have bloating, fatigue and even nausea. Chances are that these people are hypochlorhydic.

Iron deficiency anemia is a common cause of fatigue. Many times iron deficiency anemia that is not responding to iron supplementation will improve if the patient takes betaine hydrochloride (hydrochloric acid supplementation) after meals, along with the iron.

The medical model of hydrochloric acid production not being important to health and digestion is not entirely correct. There is some evidence that antacids decrease the amount of vitamin $B_{12}$ that is absorbed. Also, research indicates that people who do not produce enough stomach acid have a greater tendency to be deficient in vitamin $B_{12}$. This is especially common in the elderly. Vitamin $B_{12}$ deficiency can cause problems with poor memory, poor concentration, fatigue and even depression. There is a possibility that some patients diagnosed with having dementia or even Alzheimer's disease may actually be deficient in vitamin $B_{12}$.

Hydrochloric acid and pepsin are necessary to break protein down into individual amino acids. Without sufficient acid, protein is not completely broken down and utilized by the body. Low stomach acid causes poor protein digestion and deficiencies in the eight essential amino acids. Amino acids are the building blocks of protein. If a protein is a freight train, the amino acids are the individual cars. Essential amino acids are those that the body can't produce for itself.

The essential amino acids are very important because they are involved with the chemistry of the brain and in the endocrine system. Deficiencies in them can cause fatigue and even depression.

Tyrosine is an essential amino acid that is necessary for the formation of both thyroid hormone and epinephrine (adrenal hormone). Both of these hormones are the body's "uppers." Without sufficient tyrosine, fatigue may be a problem.

The thyroid is the body's thermostat. Thyroid hormones control the rate of metabolism, which is how fast you burn calories to produce energy. People suffering from hypothyroidism burn calories slowly. They are extremely fatigued, as well as having many other symptoms, including constipation, dry skin, brittle hair, frequent colds, obesity and trouble staying warm.

Persons with underfunctioning adrenal glands are similarly very tired and may crave salt, have dizziness when standing up suddenly, will be bothered by strong light and will have other symptoms. They sometimes have low back and medial knee pain. It is possible for a lack of hydrochloric acid to affect the adrenal and thyroid glands

Poor digestion of protein and minerals can cause people suffering from hypochlorhydra to have brittle nails and hair. It may even be responsible for hair loss. (Unfortunately, it is *not* the cause of male pattern baldness.)

The treatment for hypochlorhydia is to take betaine hydrochloride and pepsin after meals. Do not try to diagnose hypochlorhydria on your own. Taking hydrochloric acid supplements can cause problems in certain patients. Betaine hydrochloride can make ulcer patients feel much worse. Also, if you are taking any anti-inflammatory medication, such as aspirin, Motrin, Advil or any other nonsteroidal anti-inflammatory drug (NSAID), the supplement can cause an unpleasant burning sensation. NSAIDS irritate the lining of the GI tract. If the lining of the digestive tract is eroded or inflamed, from NSAID use or any other reason, hydrochloric acid supplements may cause irritation.

People suffering from a hiatal hernia will often experience burning and irritation when they take betaine hydrochloride. Normally the diaphragm helps separate the stomach from the esophagus. A hiatal hernia is a condition where the stomach protrudes above the diaphragm. This allows the acid that is in the stomach to irritate the lining of the esophagus. Symptoms can include chronic acid indigestion, nausea and even chest pain. Sometimes the pain is so severe that it can mimic a heart attack. Betaine hydrochloride may increase the pain and burning in hiatal hernia patients.

The irritation caused by betaine hydrochloride is unpleasant, but usually isn't serious. Discontinuing the supplement and taking antacids for a day or two will usually give relief. Also, just because the supplements cause irritation, doesn't mean that they are not necessary.

Many of the drugs used for depression increase the function of neurotransmitters. Essential amino acids, especially tyrosine and tryptophan, are necessary to produce these neurotransmitters. Frequently, someone who is hypochlorhydric will be depressed as well as fatigued. Supplementation with essential amino acids, along with hydrochloric acid supplementation sometimes helps these people.

One test to measure hydrochloric acid production is done by injecting histamine into the stomach and then taking samples of stomach acid through a tube every 10 minutes. The acid strength of each sample is then measured. This is an extreme measure.

There is also a machine that will test stomach acid levels, called a Heidleberg gastric analyzer. The test is easier on the patient and is usually performed right in the doctor's office. The patient swallows a capsule, which is a tiny radio transmitter. The transmitter measures the pH as it travels through the GI tract and sends the information to a receiver outside of the patient (easier for the technician to read that way).

Hypochlorhydra is fairly common. Some physicians treat it without using either of the above tests. If the patient doesn't have an ulcer or hiatal hernia, or is not taking anti-inflammatory medication, betaine hydrochloride rarely causes any trouble. Even if an unpleasant burning sensation is caused by the betaine hydrochloride, discontinuing it will usually give relief.

Hypochlorhydra can be at the root of other digestive problems. It can cause leaky gut, malabsorption and even dysbiosis.

It is worth saying a few things about patients who have gastric reflux. People are taking drugs that decrease stomach acid production. Lately the H2 receptor or histamine blockers have become available over the counter. Commercials for these products go so far as to suggest that you can take them in anticipation of eating like an idiot.

Even though these drugs are effective at reducing symptoms, they do so at a price. In patients using ranitidine (sold under the brand name Zantac) there have been cases of mental confusion, agitation, malaise, dizziness, somnolence, insomnia and vertigo. Depression and hallucinations have been reported, predominantly in severely ill elderly patients. There have been reports of arrhythmias such as tachycardia, bradycardia, atrioventricular block and premature ventricular beats. Some cases of reversible blurred vision suggestive of a change in accommodation have been reported. Rare reports of reversible involuntary motor disturbances have been received. Some patients get constipation, diarrhea, nausea/vomiting, abdominal discomfort/pain and rare reports of pancreatitis. There have been reports of joint and muscle pain and occasional reports of hepatocellular, cholestatic or mixed hepatitis. Blood count changes (leukopenia, granulocytopenia and thrombocytopenia) have occurred in a few patients. These were usually reversible. Rare cases of agranulocytosis, pancytopenia, sometimes with marrow hypoplasia, and aplastic anemia and exceedingly rare cases of acquired immune hemolytic anemia have been reported. In other words, some potential serious health problems are possible from using ranitidine. This added to the fact that these drugs interfere with the absorption of nutrients mean that the decision to go on them should not be taken lightly.

Many people who are taking antacids do not actually produce enough stomach acid. Antacids provide relief, but neutralizing stomach acid will interfere with the digestion and absorption of over 20 nutrients. This is compounded by the fact that people who inhale their food don't absorb as many nutrients as they would if they ate slowly. For years natural health care providers have been treating reflux by giving hydrochloric acid to aid digestion. It seems illogical that taking acid could relieve burning in the stomach.

But these doctors realize that the patients feel a burning sensation, not because of excess acid, but because the acid is in the wrong place.

There are a few theories about why low acid can cause burning. One is that when food enters a stomach that does not produce enough acid, the food is not digested; it rots. This unnatural breakdown of the food produces nitric and sulfuric acids. The stomach lining can tolerate a very acidic pH, but these acids also irritate and oxidize the lining—much more so than the hydrochloric acid produced by the stomach. This is not a bad idea. The normal pH of the stomach is 2; you can dissolve nails in a solution that has a pH of 2. It is very acidic; it is meant to be. The concept that people with gastric reflux produce too much acid is probably incorrect.

Another idea is that incomplete digestion creates gas and forces the acid up into the esophagus. There are two ends to the stomach, one is the esophagus and the other is the pylorus. The pylorus is the entry to the small intestine. It is a strong, muscular ring that can resist pressure much more effectively than the opening that keeps acid out of the esophagus. One theory is that the pylorus will not open unless the pH is low (acidic) enough. People who do not produce enough hydrochloric acid have trouble opening the pylorus and the contents of the stomach move back up into the esophagus.

Physicians trained in natural health care and nutrition tend to treat digestive problems like reflux by giving hydrochloric acid or digestive enzymes rather than by trying to suppress acid production. Clinically this works very well, even though there is not a lot of research to back this approach.

Occasionally a person suffering from reflux will be given hydrochloric acid and the supplement will really irritate his or her symptoms. Oddly enough, this does not mean that they do not need the acid, but rather that the lining of the esophagus and possibly the stomach is atrophied or irritated. These patients respond well when given supplementation to help heal the lining. Biotics Research makes two products that are useful for this. Gastrazyme is an extract made from cabbage; fresh cabbage juice is a traditional treatment to heal the digestive lining. In fact, if you suffer with epigastric burning, try some fresh cabbage juice, it may offer you some relief. Bio-HPF contains a number of herbs designed to keep undesirable bacteria (like heliobacter) in check, to increase mucus production, to protect the digestive lining and to heal the digestive lining.

After patients are given a supplement to promote healing, they frequently can tolerate hydrochloric acid supplements. Biotics makes a product called Hydrozyme, which has pancreatic enzymes and a very small amount of hydrochloric acid. It is a great product for gradually getting a patient used to taking hydrochloric acid supplements.

If you eat a vitamin-deficient meal, and you inhale it, you don't get much nutritional value from your meal. Also eating too rapidly causes gas, bloating and fatigue after each meal. And you wonder why you're tired.

Antacids can give relief to the problem of stomach acid irritating the esophageal lining, but they do not address the cause of the problem. Eating slowly and thoroughly chewing your food often solves the problem of acid indigestion. Often acid indigestion is triggered by certain foods. Sometimes a food allergy is involved. Identify problem foods by keeping a food diary, writing down everything that you eat. Make a note each time you get an attack of acid indigestion. If a certain food is causing the attack, you will see the pattern in your diary.

There is a chiropractic technique for hiatal hernia. It really seems to work. In the past, I've had patients describe the technique to their medical doctors. They were all told that it was ridiculous and that it couldn't work. Nonetheless, many chiropractors have given hiatal hernia sufferers relief. Maybe it's the power of our dynamic personalities creating a placebo effect. Of course, if the patient experiences relief, who cares what did it?

Patients suffering with ulcers often mistake them for acid indigestion (which is one reason you should be working with a doctor and not trying to diagnose yourself from a book). *Heliobacter pylori*, which irritates the digestive lining, is a common cause of ulcers. There is a lab test available for Heliobacter now. If Heliobacter is present, the ulcer can be treated with a course of antibiotics, or your doctor may take an herbal approach with a product like Bio-HPF.

## Dysbiosis

Residing in the large intestine are large numbers of microorganisms. Half of the volume of your stool consists of microorganisms. Some belong there and some do not. There are actually more bacterial cells in your colon than there are cells in your entire body. The bacteria belong there; they contribute to your health and well-being.

Dysbiosis refers to the absence of normal bacteria, overgrowth of pathogenic organisms or bacteria growing in an area of the digestive tract that normally has no bacteria. Perhaps the best-known form of dysbiosis is Candidiasis, which William Crook, MD, made famous in his book *The Yeast Connection*. An overgrowth of yeast, which produces toxins and undermines the health of the GI system and the immune system, is a form of dysbiosis.

Normally there are between four and seven pounds of bacteria in the colon. When the bacteria are normal and in balance, they perform many beneficial functions. Beneficial bacteria do the following:

- Produce vitamins like folic acid and $B_{12}$.
- Nourish the lining of the colon by producing butyric acid. They do this by feeding on vegetable fiber. Adequate butyric acid levels reduce the chances for colon cancer.
- Inhibit harmful bacteria.
- Break down toxins.

There are other bacteria and yeast that normally exist, but in smaller numbers. Think of the GI tract as an ecosystem, with a balance between beneficial and not-so-beneficial microorganisms. When the ecosystem is out of balance, as it is with Candidiasis, your health can be adversely affected. Harmful microorganisms do the following:

- Inhibit normal bacteria, creating deficiencies of nutrients and other problems.
- Produce toxins. Harmful bacteria create toxins and inhibit normal bacteria from detoxifying the bowel. Toxins can burden the liver and affect every function in the body.
- Hydrogenate polyunsaturated fatty acids.
- Damage the intestinal lining creating increased intestinal permeability. This eventually leads to allergies and many other chronic health problems.
- Deconjugate hormones (especially estrogen) that the liver packages up for disposal. When the body is done with hormones, they are excreted by the liver into the bile. Pathogenic bacteria put these hormones back into circulation. Often dysbiosis causes a patient to suffer from PMS because pathogenic bacteria are causing estrogen and

estrogen-like compounds that the body is eliminating to go back into circulation. This can cause a hormone imbalance. Also, there are those who think that this may increase estrogen in the body and thereby increase the chances for getting breast cancer.

Allergies, chemical sensitivities, fatigue, fibromyalgia, depression, digestive problems, skin problems, headaches, joint pain and virtually any chronic health problem can be caused by dysbiosis. These problems are the result of nutrient deficiencies, toxicity, GI irritation and challenges to the immune system.

Dysbiosis can be caused by improper eating, exposure to toxins like chemicals and heavy metals, drug therapy, poor enzyme production, nutrient deficiency or poor immune function. The huge amounts of sugar and refined carbohydrates most people eat can definitely contribute to an overgrowth of yeast in the intestine. Treating dysbiosis is important, but you also have to address the underlying cause.

### How to Determine the Presence of Dysbiosis

Diagnosis of dysbiosis can be aided by a stool analysis. By analyzing a stool sample for enzymes, various chemical components and bacterial balance, you can have an idea of how well the GI system is functioning and whether or not dysbiosis is present. It is by no means a perfect test. Parasitic infestations are often missed (about 20% of the time); only bacteria that can live in open air (around 10% of normal bowel flora) are found; and many of the indicators of enzyme function and nutrient absorption are approximations. Still, it can be a useful test.

A less expensive test is a parasite profile. It tests for yeast and parasites but does not test for enzymes and the other chemical components of the stool.

A health history and general examination can give clues as to whether or not dysbiosis is a problem. Previous eating habits, drug therapies and chemical exposures can indicate a problem with dysbiosis.

Many people are familiar with dysbiosis from Dr. William Crook's book *The Yeast Connection.* Crook's idea is that people suffering from many chronic health problems, including allergies, headaches, fatigue, body aches, asthma and skin problems, and patients who are "just plain sick" have a problem with proliferation of yeast in their large intestine.

Dysbiosis can also refer to parasites growing in the large intestine. Parasites can cause problems very similar to those that yeast causes. Because yeast is so much more common than parasites, often people go through regimens to get rid of yeast, when, in reality, their problems are caused by amoebas or other types of parasites.

Microorganisms growing where they do not belong is also a form of dysbiosis. In a sense, the word *dysbiosis* can refer to ulcers caused by Heliobacter pylori. There is a theory that Crohn's disease is caused by overgrowth of normal bacteria in the small intestine. This is dysbiosis, since bacteria do not belong in the small intestine.

**Yeast**

Candidiasis is another word for yeast infestation in the bowel. To some extent, yeast exists in everyone's digestive tract. The normal bowel flora, bacteria that belong in the bowel, keep the yeast in check. If the normal bacteria die, yeast can proliferate, causing

Candidiasis. It can lead to allergies, leaky gut and digestive disturbances. Generally Candidiasis undermines health. Patients are not only fatigued, but they may also have other symptoms such as headaches, hypoglycemia, sinus problems, irritable bowel, nausea and other digestive problems, joint pain, rashes, hives, and other skin problems. Smoke and fumes often bother them. They often suffer from the just-plain-sick syndrome—feeling miserable, but unable to get a definite diagnosis from allopathic physicians.

Candida patients tend to feel worse in damp and dark places. This is because mold grows in moist dark places and Candida patients tend to be sensitive to mold. Also, smoke and perfume can cause a flare-up of symptoms. Many people who now have a problem with yeast and mold often have a history of eating a lot of refined food or frequent treatment with antibiotics. Eating a highly refined diet, with lots of sugar and refined white flour, nourishes the yeast and kills the normal bacteria. Frequent use of antibiotics can lead to yeast proliferation in the large intestine.

Antibiotics kill normal bowel bacteria, but leave the yeast unmolested. Repeated ear infections as a child, antibiotic therapy for acne as a teenager, recurrent bladder or sinus infections or bouts of strep throat are common reasons for antibiotic therapy. Many people who do not now enjoy good health had a period in their life when they took a lot of antibiotics.

The large intestine has wildlife in it, much like a forest or any other ecosystem. If the wolves are killed off, the forest becomes overgrown with deer and rabbits. In the intestine, if the normal bacteria are killed off, the intestine becomes overgrown with yeast and pathogenic bacteria.

Also, repeated bouts of antibiotic therapy tend to create *super bugs*, or bacteria that are antibiotic resistant. Antibiotics, while curing the immediate problem, predispose patients to future infections by disturbing the normal floral balance and by creating antibiotic-resistant strains of bacteria. This is on top of the fact that frequent use of antibiotics can cause yeast overgrowth in the large intestine.

Yeasts are one-celled organisms. They are like little chemical factories. They feed on carbohydrates, especially sugars. They release waste material, which contributes to the taste of foods like cheddar cheese, vinegar and beer. In the intestines, the waste products of the yeast can create problems. They irritate the intestinal lining and they kill normal bacteria, causing leaky gut and making dysbiosis worse. The chemical toxins from the yeast are also absorbed by the body and can cause intolerance for smoke, perfumes and other chemicals by overloading the body's mechanism to remove them. They burden the liver.

Yeast and their chemical waste products eventually challenge the integrity of the intestinal wall leading to a condition known as leaky gut. This can cause allergies. In leaky gut, the intestine is not an effective barrier. Material in the intestines is technically outside of the body, with the intestinal wall acting as a barrier between it and the bloodstream. In leaky gut, the intestinal wall's effectiveness as a barrier is compromised and things that belong outside of the body are absorbed into the bloodstream.

Much of the therapy for Candidiasis concentrates on killing the yeast. Some physicians merely have patients take Nystatin to kill the yeast; *and* they are on a very strict diet. Sometimes yeast proliferation can be brought under control without as heavy-handed an approach as some of the antiyeast programs. Taking Nystatin long-term is not usually necessary. In fact, many patients effectively handle their yeast problem without the use of drugs.

One problem with taking Nystatin long-term is that not all strains of Candida are sensitive to it. Also, yeast can mutate and develop tolerance to antifungal substances. Anything that you take to kill yeast will eventually lose its effectiveness. Another reason that Nystatin is not always effective is the fact that yeast can exist in several forms, some of which are more virulent than others. In its more virulent state, yeast can invade the wall of the intestine, making it harder to treat. Nystatin, which does not get into the bloodstream, may not be effective. Nyzoral, a drug that does enter the blood stream is sometimes used to kill the more virulent form of yeast. There are herbs and other natural substances that will also kill the more tenacious form of yeast. These include caprillic acid, undecenoic acid, grapefruit seed extract and garlic.

An effective strategy for bringing Candidiasis under control is to take one of these substances for about a month and then switch to another one. Garlic and undecenoic acid are also absorbed into the bloodstream and can kill the more virulent form of yeast.

There is a product made from oregano, called A.D.P. It is manufactured by Biotics Research. Clinically, this substance seems to be a very effective antifungal. It also seems to kill much more than just yeast. It can kill pathogenic bacteria and some parasites.

If you take A.D.P., as with any antiyeast regimen, replacing the normal bacteria is very important. Take acidophilus and bifidus bacteria for at least 60 days after you finish taking A.D.P. These substances nourish normal bacteria, without feeding yeast or pathogenic bacteria. Strictly avoid refined carbohydrates like sugar and white flour. Sugar and starch feed yeast and suppress the growth of normal bacteria.

There are many people who are given a diagnosis of Candidiasis who are avoiding yeast. This isn't necessary unless they are also allergic to yeast.

Yeast overgrowth in the intestine and yeast allergy are not the same things; however, they can exist together.

In treating Candidiasis, it is more important to treat the body that has the yeast, rather than just treating the yeast. Frequently patients undergoing treatment for Candida will still be experiencing symptoms and they will interpret those symptoms as, "The yeast is still there." In reality, the symptoms are from nutrient deficiencies, leaky gut or allergies. Dealing with all of the health issues is a much more effective way of treating Candidiasis patients than becoming obsessed with killing the yeast. Sometimes the patient responds to these antiyeast regimens, but the Candidiasis keeps coming back. These patients may have problems with heavy metals, adrenals, hypochlorhydra, the immune system or other underlying problem. Candida is both a cause and an effect: It can cause many symptoms, but it often is the result of some other health problem. It is much wiser to treat the patient who has the Candida rather than to treat the Candida that has the patient.

In a healthy bowel, the normal bacteria keep the yeast in check. Taking lactobacillus and bifidus bacteria is helpful, but often these organisms don't survive in a yeast-infested gut. Changing the environment of the bowel will promote the growth of normal bacteria and keep the yeast in check.

Something as simple as eating vegetables will help balance the bowel flora, eliminating yeast and nurturing the normal bacteria, which feed on vegetable fiber. Make a raw, chopped salad two or three times each day. Take any raw vegetables that you like and chop them in a food processor. You can season them with salt, pepper, oil and lemon. It is tasty and good for your digestion. The vegetable fiber helps nourish the healthful bacteria, the fiber will decrease absorption of toxins and the vegetables themselves contain phytochemicals, carotenes and folic acid that are all good for the health of the intestinal lining.

Strictly avoid refined sugar and white flour. This is vital. If yeast is a problem, you will not return to health if you persist in eating refined foods. Yeast feeds on carbohydrate and really thrives on refined carbohydrate.

Vitamin supplementation is also important, since many of the symptoms suffered by Candida patients are the result of nutrient deficiency. Everyone is unique. There is no single Candida nutrient program. A good multiple vitamin, some vitamin B complex and vitamin C are a good start. Biotin, a B vitamin, suppresses yeast growth and helps normal bacteria to grow. Trace minerals are especially important. Sensitivity to smoke and perfume is one of the more common symptoms of Candida patients. Taking a trace mineral, molybdenum, often alleviates this symptom; sometimes taking vitamin $B_{12}$ also helps.

Testing stool samples for yeast is a good way to monitor the efficacy of your treatment. Your health care provider trained in nutrition can help you to determine if you need to be tested. Testing can also keep you from persisting in taking herbs or even drugs unnecessarily.

Candidiasis is a controversial subject. Many physicians don't believe that it even exists. A recent study in a respected medical journal had subjects suspected of suffering from Candidiasis taking Nystatin. No other type of therapy, nutritional supplementation or diet was included in the study. The study concluded that Nystatin was of no value to these patients. Of course, the doctors who ran this study are now gearing up to study the phenomena of frogs that are hard of hearing and their inability to jump.

Another controversy is how important is it to kill the yeast? Yeast is an opportunistic organism; in other words, it does not proliferate unless conditions are right. It may not be necessary to try to eliminate the yeast, but rather improve other aspects of the digestive and immune system. Sometimes it is best to treat digestive problems from north to south; in other words, make sure there is adequate enzyme or hydrochloric acid production in the stomach before you worry about what is going on in the colon. Many times people who have a problem with Candida do so because of other health issues. Stress causes an individual to produce a lot of cortisol, which feeds yeast. Chemical and heavy metal toxicity can also be underlying causes of yeast overgrowth. Some doctors who deal in natural health will take the approach of simply changing the diet and fixing some of these other health issues, letting the Candidiasis resolve itself over time. Find a health care provider trained in nutrition and natural health care to help find the right approach to this problem.

The following dietary advice will help bring Candida under control. Think of this as a start to balancing the flora in your digestive system.

**Lifestyle Changes for Candida Patients**

- *Eat two, large chopped salads each day:* Normal flora feed on vegetable fiber. Eating the chopped salads will help normal, beneficial bacteria to thrive.
- *Avoid refined carbohydrates:* These feed yeast and will prolong treatment. Sometimes it is necessary to limit carbohydrates. Some practitioners limit carbohydrate consumption to 60–80 grams of carbohydrate per day. Others use allergy diets. Elaine Gottschall's Specific Carbohydrate Diet is actually a pretty good diet—even though it is not specifically for yeast.
- *Chew your food thoroughly:* This improves digestion, breaking down food particles and mixing

them with salivary enzymes. The better your digestion, the easier it is to treat dysbiosis.

- ***Don't eat a lot of meat:*** You don't have to avoid it completely (unless allergies are at issue). Eating too much meat can feed certain species of undesirable bacteria. Your doctor will make specific dietary recommendations.
- ***Avoid dairy products.***
- ***Eat plenty of raw vegetables:*** Raw foods contain enzymes and aid digestion. Vegetable fiber helps nourish normal bacteria. In fact, it is so important, it bears repeating: Make a large, finely chopped salad twice each day. (Oh yes, and eat it!)
- ***Find and eliminate hidden food sensitivities:*** Avoiding hidden allergens can reduce the burden on the immune system and make it easier for the body to resist dysbiotic organisms. Try the Healing Diet first. It is usually very good for keeping Candida under control; it is very nutrient-rich. It is just as important, if not more important, to consume nutrient-rich food as it is to avoid foods that aggravate the condition.

### *A complete program to control dysbiosis will address all of the following:*

- Treat the upper GI, making sure that the early phases of digestion are properly working (use of enzymes, hydrochloric acid etc.).
- Kill the offending organism. You don't necessarily need a drug here; an oregano extract (like ADP), garlic, caprillic acid or other substance that your health care provider recommends will do just fine.
- Heal the GI lining. Biotics Research makes a good product for this—IPS (stands for intestinal permeability support). Other things that will help to heal the GI tract include aloe vera, glutamine and folic acid.

135

- Replace the normal flora. Take acidophilus and bifidus; your health care provider can help you find a good product and select the right dosage.

Effectively treating Candidiasis involves a multifaceted approach. Modern medicine, with its propensity toward single-element treatments, tends to disbelieve the idea that *Candida albicans* can cause systemic disease. Of course at one time, respected physicians thought that Pasteur's ideas were a lot of nonsense.

**Parasites**

Parasitic infection can lead to the following symptoms: chronic fatigue, abdominal pain and cramps, anorexia, autoimmune disease, distention, fever, food allergy, gastritis, inflammatory bowel disease, leaky gut, irregular bowel movements, irritable bowel disease, low back pain, itching anus, rashes, hives, weight loss, arthritis, bloody stools, colitis, Crohn's disease, diarrhea, dysentery, flatulence, foul-smelling stools, headaches, malabsorption, vomiting and even depression. Many times patients who are suspected of having Cadidiasis actually have parasites.

One of the most common misconceptions about parasites is the idea that they are extremely rare. They are much more common than most people realize. Many physicians think of parasitic infection as a disease of the tropics or of the third world. Although parasites are more common in the tropics, they also exist in the United States. We have truly become a world village. People from the tropics, and from the rest of the planet, live in the United States. We import produce from all around the world. People can travel halfway around the world in a single day. People from the United States regularly go to the tropics. This blending of populations includes blending of microbial populations. We are no longer protected from parasitic infection by winter and distance.

Estimates vary, but between 15% and 30% of Americans have a parasitic infection. Great Smokies Diagnostic Laboratory reports that 30% of the samples it tests contain parasites. This number may be higher than the general population since people tend to send samples to Great Smokies when they have gastrointestinal complaints.

Parasites that infect the human intestinal tract are either protozoa (one-celled organisms) or helminths (worms). They are found by testing stool samples. Even laboratories that specialize in testing stool samples, like Meridian Labs, Doctor's Data and Great Smokies, can miss finding a parasite, although they do a better job than most hospitals. Frequently, several types of samples are used, including samples of regular bowel movements, bowel movements taken after using a laxative (purged stool sample) and by swabbing the area around the anus (to find eggs left by worms). Finding parasites is very difficult. The technician literally has to sort through poop to find something microscopic in size. (I don't know what these labs pay, but these guys can't be making enough money.)

Most hospital labs do not take parasites very seriously. You may be asked if you've been to the tropics. You may tell them no, but you've been to Jamaica Joe's Cajun Sushi Bar on the West Side of Chicago and that you've had gas and diarrhea for the last eight months. Your vinyl upholstery is starting to crack and blister, and no one will sit in a car with you. In fact, on the way to the doctor, the cab driver paid you to get out. The lab may reluctantly agree to take your sample, since they've just gotten a patient from Jamaica Joe's who's been on IV fluids for the last three weeks. They test your stool, without a purged sample or a peri-anal swab, and it comes out negative. You are given some Kaopectate, a clothespin for your spouse's nose and the doctor's condolences.

Just because a laboratory didn't find a parasite doesn't mean that one doesn't exist. There is a certain amount of skill required in preparing and reading the sample. Taking different types of stool samples is also very important. Sometimes several stool samples test negative before a parasite is actually found. It is best to use a laboratory that specializes in finding parasites and that takes parasitic infection seriously.

While it is true that the most common symptoms of parasitic infection are abdominal pain, gas and diarrhea, it is possible to have a parasitic infection without these symptoms. A person infected with parasites may simply be fatigued or depressed. Sometimes the parasite only causes gastrointestinal problems at one stage of its life cycle, so that the patient only experiences gas, abdominal pain or diarrhea occasionally.

**Bowel Ecology**

Good bowel ecology is necessary if you are to have enough energy. Poor bowel ecology can lead not only to fatigue, but to many other health problems as well. Even diseases like rheumatoid arthritis, ankylosing spondylitis and other autoimmune diseases seem to be caused by bowel problems. Individuals with these diseases form antibodies to bacteria in the intestine. These antibodies attack the individual's own tissue, creating the autoimmune disease.

Normal flora in the large intestine is necessary to keep yeast and pathogenic bacteria in check. Normal flora competes with yeast and pathogens for nutrients, and normal flora produces natural antibiotics. Normal flora also breaks down toxins produced by the yeast and pathogens.

The environment of the colon determines what kind of microorganisms will live there. The pH, fiber content, enzymes and cell integrity of the bowel are very important. Diets that are low in fiber and high in sugar and fat can also create an environment for dysbiosis. Yeast and pathogenic bacteria will thrive at the expense of normal bacteria. Drugs, especially antibiotics, steroids and alcohol can contribute to yeast overgrowth, as can stress, cortisol, excess bile production and heavy metals.

Poor bowel ecology, or dysbiosis, causes an increase in toxic chemicals in the bowel, such as ammonia, phenols, amines, nitrites and aldehydes. The toxic chemicals of the pathogens further suppress the growth of normal bacteria and irritate the lining of the intestine. Pathogenic bacteria can even increase estrogen levels and thereby play a role in PMS and breast cancer.

The loss of normal bacteria also causes a loss of nutrients that they produce, including vitamin $B_{12}$, vitamin K and other substances such as short-chain fatty acids. These are meant to nourish the lining of the large intestine. The result can be fatigue, anemia, neurological problems, easy bruising and leaky gut.

In a dysbiotic bowel more ammonia is absorbed than in a normal bowel. Ammonia inhibits oxidative metabolism in the brain. Absorption of ammonia and other toxic chemicals can lead to a deep fatigue that many patients describe as being like a hangover. These patients are so fatigued, that no amount of sleep seems to make them feel better. They have a foggy feeling and poor concentration. Dr. Theron Randolph coined the term *brain fag*. Dr. Randolph wasn't homophobic, *fag* is actually short for fatigue. To avoid confusion, some clinical ecologists use the term *brain fog*.

Brain fog is a common complaint of patients with food allergies, dysbiosis and chemical sensitivity. It is primarily caused by toxicity. Toxins from yeast, pathogenic bacteria, parasites, toxins absorbed from leaky gut and chemical debris from an overworked immune system can all cause brain fog. If you've ever had a bad hangover, you have a good idea of what brain fog feels like.

Dysbiosis can also refer to normal bacteria living in the small intestine, where they don't belong. There is some speculation that Crohn's disease is caused by overgrowth of normal bacteria in the small intestine.

Crohn's disease, or regional ileitis, is an inflammatory disease of the small intestine. Sections of the small intestine become irritated. As the inflammation persists, the intestine narrows and becomes hard. These patients often suffer from severe abdominal cramping and other bowel disturbances. Sometimes the bowel becomes so narrow and loses so much of its elasticity that sections of it must be removed surgically.

Crohn's disease is very complicated. In some cases, mycobacterium have been involved. These patients also have increased intestinal permeability (leaky gut—see the next section). Their white blood cells often overreact to *Candida albicans* and to normal flora. They are often deficient in zinc, selenium, magnesium, and pretty near everything else. Supplementation is often beneficial to these patients.

Crohn's patients often benefit from a diet that is low in sugars. Also, eating meals that consist of a single food is beneficial. Finding and avoiding food allergens helps to alleviate the symptoms of Crohn's disease. Gluten is a common allergen that Crohn's sufferers react to. I remember one Crohn's patient that called and couldn't get into the office for a while. He asked what he could do for himself in the mean time. I told him to avoid wheat and refined sugar. I never saw him as a patient. I ran into him a few months later and he said that he never came into the office because his Crohn's went into remission. Obviously not every patient with Crohn's will get this kind of result just from giving up wheat and sugar, but it does happen.

Refined sugar is an aggravating factor for Crohn's. One study that looked at the effect of refined sugar on Crohn's disease was canceled because the sugar exacerbated the symptoms of so many people participating in the study.

Many Crohn's patients benefit from a diet known as the Specific Carbohydrate Diet, presented in Elaine Gottschall's book *Ending the Vicious Cycle*. The diet limits the type of carbohydrates patients can eat. They are allowed no complex carbohydrates (starches, including those in whole grain). Fruit is permissible, refined sugar is not. Its goal is to limit microbial growth in the intestine. No grains, potatoes, soybeans or chick peas are permitted. If you suffer from Crohn's disease or ulcerative colitis, this book is worth getting. The diet doesn't cure everyone, but those it does help often have a *permanent* remission of symptoms, without having to stay on the diet forever.

Elaine Gottschall believes that the problem begins with eating too much complex carbohydrate too quickly. The enzymes from the pancreas do not do an adequate job of digesting these carbohydrates, so they pass into the intestine without being completely digested. Because they are not digested, they foster the growth of undesirable bacteria. The undesirable bacteria cause the food to rot in the intestine. The rotting food irritates the cells of the intestine, decreasing their enzyme output, further increasing the amount of food available for the bacteria, causing them to grow, creating further irritation, less enzyme production etc. It creates a vicious cycle.

The diet doesn't work on every case of Crohn's, but it works on some. Gottschall's program can be improved by taking enzymes with your meals, general nutrients and something to help the intestinal wall to heal (like IPS from Biotics Research).

Ulcerative colitis is similar to Crohn's disease. Crohn's is a disease of the small intestine, while ulcerative colitis is a disease of the large intestine. These patients often have amoebic infection (parasites). Frequently, they will have had amoebic dysentery in the past. A pathogenic bacteria known as *Clostridium dificile* is often involved. Testing the stool for parasites or pathogenic bacteria is advisable. Patients often do well by giving up dairy products. High doses of fish oil sometimes help to control the inflammation of ulcerative colitis. Eighteen capsules per day of Max-EPA (fish oil) have been given in clinical trials with encouraging results.

Another clinical trial involved treating ulcerative colitis patients by killing all of the bowel floras with massive doses of antibiotics. The patients were then given a mixture of normal bowel flora. Eighty-six percent of these patients went into remission. This is not a practical treatment, but it does show a definite connection between dysbiosis and ulcerative colitis.

There may be a variety of causes for diseases like Crohn's and ulcerative colitis. The specific carbohydrate diet will help many of these patients, but not all. Finding allergies, balancing bowel flora, killing pathogens, and nutrient supplementation can improve the results gotten from the diet. Of course it is best to get help from a trained professional.

Crohn's disease and ulcerative colitis are just two examples of diseases that may be caused by dysbiosis. There is evidence to show that psoriatic arthritis, ankylosing spondylitis, psoriasis, eczema and rheumatoid arthritis are also linked to dysbiosis.

Problems with the gut flora can go beyond fatigue. Skin trouble, arthritis, digestive problems, autoimmune diseases, PMS and even cancer can be linked to dysbiosis.

## Leaky Gut

Material in the digestive tract is still technically outside of the body. The cells lining the GI system break the material down and selectively absorb nutrients. These cells act as a barrier between the bloodstream and the digestive material. Alcohol, drugs, a highly refined diet, environmental poisons and toxins resulting from dysbiosis all irritate the cells lining the intestinal tract. Over time the cells become ineffective barriers against toxic molecules, undigested protein and even microorganisms. If the situation continues unchecked, large molecules, which would normally remain in the intestine, enter the bloodstream. Once in the bloodstream, these large molecules are not recognized as food, but as foreign invaders, triggering a response from the immune system. This is known as *leaky gut*.

Protein is important to the immune system. Proteins are large molecules, much like a freight train. The train is made up of smaller molecules, analogous to the cars of the train. These smaller molecules are called amino acids. There are 22 of them. Eight of the 22 are essential; they have to be provided externally because the body can't manufacture them. In a healthy digestive system, any protein eaten is absorbed as individual amino acids. If it is not completely broken down, a healthy intestine will keep it out of the bloodstream. In leaky gut, incompletely digested protein, called peptides, are absorbed.

Peptides are groups of amino acids linked together. They are large enough to be noticed by the immune system, which works by recognizing protein that doesn't belong in the body. Protein provides the

143

structure of the cell; that is, its framework. It is very much like the 2 x 4 studs that make up the frame of a house.

The structure of invading organisms, like viruses and bacteria, has its own protein frame. Your immune system recognizes the difference between the framework of your own cells and the framework of the invaders' cells.

When an invader is recognized, the cells of the immune system attack it. They release chemicals, like histamines and kinins, to destroy the invaders. White blood cells, known as phagocytes, absorb the invaders. There is chemical warfare, producing free radicals. Symptoms experienced when the body is sick, such as fever, runny nose, muscle aches and other symptoms, are usually due to the actions of the immune system.

When a peptide is absorbed by someone suffering from leaky gut the immune system doesn't know the difference between the peptide and an invading virus. Chemical warfare begins. The nose runs, sinuses fill up and the sufferer becomes fatigued. An allergy develops. If long-term exposure occurs, the individual may suffer from asthma, migraines, severe fatigue, colitis, immune suppression, frequent infections, eczema and other skin problems or just about any chronic health problem you can name.

People who suffer with these symptoms have many allergies. Some of the allergies they are aware of, others, they are not. Also, those who suffer from the just-plain-sick syndrome usually have some kind of digestive problem. A combination of leaky gut and hypochlorhydra is very common. Hypochlorhydra causes incomplete protein digestion, thus forming many peptides. It can also cause an imbalance in the bacterial flora, leading to leaky gut. Leaky gut causes the peptides to be absorbed, putting the immune system in disarray.

Leaky gut may partially explain the connection between autoimmune diseases and problems with the digestive tract. Autoimmune diseases often result from immune system responses that have gotten out of control and begun to attack the body's own cells. For instance, some evidence exists that some cases of rheumatoid arthritis are the result of the body being hypersensitive to a pathogen in the bowel. The immune system attacks the bacteria, but the bacteria have similarities to their own cartilage. The immune system then attacks the joint cartilage, resulting in red, swollen, painful and distorted joints.

## A Few Final Words about Digestion

You can see how complicated finding and treating problems with digestion can be. It really is best to get professional help, but the more you know about these issues, the better. Knowing what the problem is enables you to make intelligent choices about your diet and begin to bring the problem under control. If supplementation is necessary, it is best to get the help of a trained professional.

*Is Hypochlorhydara a problem?* Ask yourself the following questions:

- Do you bloat or become fatigued within an hour of a meal?
- Do you have gas (belching) frequently?
- Do you have reflux symptoms more than twice each week?
- Do you dislike meat (or are a vegetarian for other than moral reasons)?
- Do you feel better if you do not eat a large meal?
- Do your fingernails break easily?
- Does taking vitamins upset your stomach?

If you answered yes to more than three of these questions, you may need betaine hydrochloride or pancreatic enzymes to help you to digest your meals. Other clues include the lack of desire to eat in the morning and bad breath. One way to distinguish if you need betaine hydrochloride instead of pancreatic enzymes is to use the Ridler reflexes. There are points on either side of the xiphoid process (the pointy bone at the tip of the sternum), right where the bottom of the rib cage meets the sternum. If the point on the right is tender, there is a likely need for pancreatic enzymes. If the point on the left is tender, there is a likely need for betaine hydrochloride.

A health care professional may use the Heidleberg gastric analyzer to measure stomach acid. This test uses a radio transmitter to measure the pH of the stomach. (The patient swallows a capsule that transmits to a receiver that the doctor reads.) Other practitioners may use muscle testing, neurolingual testing or even extrapolate results from a blood chemistry or a stool test.

*Is Candidiasis a problem?* Ask yourself the following questions:

- Do you eat refined sugar or starch at most meals?
- Have you had broad spectrum antibiotics more than once, or have you gone on tetracycline (e.g.,. acne treatment) or other antibiotic more than four times in you lifetime?
- If you are a woman, do you get vaginal yeast infections?
- Do you have symptoms or feel worse when you are in a moldy or musty place?
- Does smoke or perfume bother you?
- Do you frequently get lower bowel gas?

- Do you have a lot of chronic health problems like eczema, digestive problems (gas, constipation, diarrhea), headaches, fatigue, allergies etc?

If you answered yes to three or more of these questions, there is a good chance that Candida is contributing to your health problems.

## ALLERGIES

An allergy is an inappropriate response to an innocuous substance. Most people think of an allergic reaction as being sudden and severe. You break out in hives after eating strawberries; you smell ragweed and have a sneezing fit; or your eyes itch and water when you're exposed to dust. Allergic responses, however, are not always so obvious.

Allergic reactions are many and varied. The sudden onset of symptoms is only one way to react. If you are mildly allergic to something, it may take several exposures in a short period of time to evoke a response. For example, a milk allergy may give you sinus problems, but if you only have a little milk during the course of a week, you may not experience any symptoms. If, however, you have a lot of milk on a given day or have milk several days in a row, and your sinuses begin to fill up, you may never make the connection between your symptoms and the allergy.

There is another type of allergic reaction, known as the addictive allergy. This is an allergic reaction where you crave the food to which you are allergic. You crave the substance like an alcoholic craves alcohol. In fact, Dr. Theron Randolph, a noted allergist and pioneer in the field of environmental medicine, calls alcoholism the ultimate food allergy.

Randolph was one of the first, if not the first doctor, to espouse the idea of an addictive allergy. He did so in the face of criticism from his colleagues. His contribution to health care and his courage should put his name among the likes of Pasteur in the history of medicine. One of Randolph's books, *An Alternative Approach to Allergies*, is particularly worth getting. It will cover the topic of allergies in much more depth than these few pages.

People with addictive allergies eat the food that they are addicted to every day. They usually don't even know that they are allergic to that food. In fact, when told that they may be allergic to a favorite food, they are incredulous. "I can't be allergic to *that*, I eat it every day." The real tip-off to an addictive allergy is that the patient is very distressed at the idea of giving up that particular food, much the same way that an alcoholic is distressed at the idea of giving up alcohol.

People with addictive allergies suffer from a wide variety of symptoms, including fatigue, obesity, overeating, chronic sinus problems, repeated infections, hives, rashes, acne or other skin problems, digestive problems, headaches, anxiety depression, joint pain or hypoglycemia. Even gallstones may be caused by allergies. Instead of having sudden and severe symptoms, people with addictive allergies have chronic problems that they seldom associate with their allergy.

These are often patients who are just plain sick and go from doctor to doctor and receive little help. Frequently a doctor will tell them that it is all in their head. It is the ultimate medical ego trip, "If I can't fix you, you must be a hypochondriac." Along with all of the physical misery these patients suffer, sometimes they also begin to believe that they are crazy.

There is a link between allergies and digestive problems. One clinical study showed that children with giardiasis (an amebic parasite) produced more allergic antigens than children who were not infected with the parasite. Leaky gut, which can cause allergies by allowing foreign material into the bloodstream, can be caused by parasites.

Allergic reactions can also cause leaky gut. It's a chicken-and-egg situation. Which came first, the allergy or the digestive problem? Both problems need to be addressed. You need to know what your allergens are, and you need to address any digestive problems that are present.

The concept of addictive allergy is still not widely accepted. Many allergists only believe in immediate allergic reactions. However, when an addictive allergy is identified, and that substance is avoided, the patient often improves dramatically.

Some of the more common foods Americans are allergic to include the following: corn, dairy, wheat, yeast, eggs, citrus, nightshade vegetables (tomato, pepper, potato and eggplant), coffee, chocolate and soy. Finding foods that you have addictive allergies to may be tricky.

The lab tests for allergies are far from perfect. The traditional scratch tests are very inaccurate. In fact, according to Dr. Marshal Mandell, they may be as much as 80% inaccurate. Blood tests for allergies are available. The RAST test, which is an acronym for radioallerosorbent test, is one where the blood is exposed to an allergen and the immune response is noted. There are inaccuracies with RAST testing, and it also does not indicate the severity of the allergic response. This is a standard test performed by most hospital labs.

One test worth mentioning here is the ELISA/ACT test. It does measure the severity of the immune response. It is advanced testing for delayed reactions (often called *hidden allergies*) to foods and chemicals. It can be done through testing of the body's immune reactive white cells (lymphocytes). ELISA/ACT tests all delayed pathways and can test for reactions to over 300 substances. This test was developed by Dr. Russell Jaffe and is available from Serammune Physician's Labs at 800-553-5472. You can call them and find a physician who uses their services.

One of the most effective ways of finding allergies is to fast for four days. When you begin eating, introduce only one food each day and watch for a reaction. This approach should be taken only under a doctor's care. You'd be surprised how severely you can react to a food that you used to eat every day and thought was harmless. Another way to find hidden allergies is with the Coca Pulse Test.

### Coca Pulse Test Procedure (To Find Hidden Food Sensitivities)

1. Establish a baseline pulse by counting the pulse for a full minute before trying a particular food.
2. Put a food in your mouth (on the tongue). It must not be swallowed. Taste it for at least one minute.
3. Retake the pulse while the food remains in your mouth. Take the pulse for a full minute. A change of four or more is considered a sensitive reaction. The greater the degree of allergenicity, the higher the pulse will be.
4. Spit out the tested ingredient (do not swallow it) and rinse your mouth with water; retake the pulse. When it returns to baseline, another food can be tested. This test may not be valid if you are taking a drug that controls the heart rate, such as a calcium channel blocker or a beta-blocker.

There are several rules for accurate pulse testing.

• Because accuracy is important, the pulse must be measured for one full minute.
• If the pulse count when standing is greater than that when sitting, it is a positive indication of food or

environmental sensitivity.

- If the pulse count is measured at least 14 times each day, and if the daily maximal pulse rate is constant (within one or two beats) for three days in succession, it indicates that all food sensitivities have been avoided on those days.
- If the ingestion of a frequently eaten food causes no acceleration of the pulse rate (at least six beats above your estimated normal maximum) that food can be tentatively considered nonsensitive.
- The pulse reaction to an inhaled allergen (particularly dust mites) is more likely to be of shorter duration than a reaction to a major food allergen.
- Pulse rates that are not more than six beats above the estimated normal daily maximum should not be blamed on a recently eaten food but on an inhalant or recurrent reaction.
- If the lowest pulse rate does not regularly occur before rising, after the night's rest, but at some other time in the day, it usually indicates sensitivity to dust, dust mites or something in the sleeping environment.

One of the pioneers in the field of food allergy, Dr. Herbert Rinkel, discovered the hidden allergy phenomena quite by accident. Dr. Rinkel and his family ate eggs every day when he was in medical school. His father, a Kansas farmer, sent him a gross of eggs each week to help him hold expenses down.

Dr. Rinkel had a chronic runny nose, and had tried various changes in his diet to get rid of it. He did not consider eggs to be part of his problem because eating large numbers of eggs made no difference in his symptoms. Dr. Rinkel was at a party, and after having no eggs for five days, had a piece of cake. The cake was made with eggs and he immediately collapsed. This is exactly how people with addictive allergies react after removing a substance for several days and then reintroducing it.

Dr. Rinkel's original attitude that the eggs were not part of his problem is the exact attitude most allergists take toward allergy, even today. Eating eggs while in the addictive state makes no changes in the symptoms; therefore, eggs are not the problem. This is the key to the controversy between clinical ecologists, who believe that many, if not most, chronic symptoms can be caused by allergies; and traditional Western-trained doctors, who believe that allergies result in sudden, definite reactions.

If you suspect that you have food allergies, you could go to a doctor who is recommended by the American Academy of Environmental Medicine. These are doctors who understand the value of natural therapies and are familiar with the concept of addictive allergies. The Academy's number is 303-622-9755.

Treatment for allergies includes inoculating small amounts of the antigen (substance that causes the allergy) into the body, or placing a dilute solution of the offending agent under the tongue. Simple avoidance is one approach; you find out what you are allergic to and avoid it. Avoidance becomes difficult if you are allergic to a great many things. Another approach to food allergies is to avoid the substances to which you are allergic and follow the rotary diversified diet, also called the rotation diet. The rotation diet is recommended because eating the same foods over and over again can create new allergies. Sometimes the food can be reintroduced into the diet after a six-week avoidance period. Sometimes patients have so many allergies that total avoidance is impossible. These patients need to follow the rotary diet and avoid the substances to which they react the most.

If you have not identified your food allergies, you can still go on the rotation diet. In fact, it is a way to help your allergies without doing anything that may cause you harm.

During the rotation diet, you may begin to discover which foods upset you. You may become fatigued or feel bloated after a meal containing allergens. You may really miss the allergic food on the three days that you don't eat it. Your pulse may speed up after eating a food that you are allergic to.

Here is a sample of the rotary diversified diet. There is a bigger selection of foods available. This is just a sample to give you an idea how the diet works.

| Day | Breakfast | Lunch | Dinner |
|---|---|---|---|
| 1 | Oatmeal | Avocado, tuna | Turkey, green beans |
| 2 | Melon | Pork, cabbage | Halibut, carrots |
| 3 | Eggs (omelet with spinach, onion) | Lentils | Salmon, spinach |
| 4 | Quinoa | Swordfish, Broccoli | Beef, broccoli |

You can make the diet more alkaline by ensuring that the volume of fruit and vegetable is greater that that of meat or grain. Also avoid meat/grain combinations and fruit/grain combinations.

In the rotary diet, no food can be eaten more than every four days. Foods in the same family cannot be eaten more than every two days. Onion and asparagus are both in the lily family. If you have onion on Monday, you can't have asparagus on Tuesday.

Combination foods are a problem. Mayonnaise, for example, has dairy, eggs, yeast, soy and apple (from cider vinegar). You could not have beef, chicken, strawberries, beans or mushrooms the day after you had mayonnaise. Strawberries are related to apples; beans are related to soy; mushrooms are related to yeast (which is used to ferment the vinegar); chicken is related to egg; and beef is related to dairy.

A partial list of food families is shown below. This is just to give you an idea of some of the relationships. The list is derived from the one in Theron Randolph's book *An Alternative Approach to Allergies.* The list in Randolph's book was originally printed in "Coping With Your Allergies" by Natalie Golos and Frances Golos Golbitz. These sources will give you a complete listing of the foods and their families.

**Fungi:** Yeasts and molds, citric acid (a yeast by-product), mushrooms.

**Grass:** Barley, corn, rice, oat, sugar cane, wheat.

**Lily:** Aloe, asparagus, chives, garlic, leek, onion.

**Goosefoot:** Beet, chard, spinach, sugar beet.

**Laurel:** Avocado, bay leaf, cinnamon, sassafras.

**Mustard:** Broccoli, Brussel sprouts, cabbage, cauliflower, collards, horseradish, kale, kohlrabi, mustard greens, mustard seed, radish, rutabaga, turnip, watercress.

**Rose:** Apple, pear, quince, rosehips, almond, apricot, cherry, peach, nectarine, plum, most berries (but not cranberries or blueberries).

**Legume:** Alfalfa, fava beans, lima beans, mung beans, navy beans, string beans, kidney beans, black-eyed peas, carob, lentil, pea, peanut, soybean.

**Carrot:** Carrot, anise, caraway, celery, coriander, cumin, dill, fennel, parsley, parsnip.

**Mint:** Basil, marjoram, oregano, peppermint, rosemary, sage, spearmint, thyme.

**Potato:** Eggplant, bell peppers, chili peppers, cayenne, paprika, potato, tomato, tobacco.

**Composite:** Chicory, dandelion, endive, escarole, globe artichoke, Jerusalem artichoke, lettuce, Romaine, safflower oil, sunflower, tarragon.

**Gourd:** Melons, cucumber, squashes, zucchini.
**Bovine:** Beef, dairy, buffalo, goat, sheep.

The rotation diet is only one approach to food allergies. People suffering from allergies are not necessarily doomed to a life of avoidance. Since nutritional deficiency contributes to allergies, proper nutritional supplementation can help you to tolerate the things to which you are sensitive.

There are many well-documented cases of people who have been exposed to chemicals and developed many sensitivities. Physicians using natural health care are well aware of the fact that these patients respond to vitamin therapy. Vitamin C can reduce histamine levels. Trace minerals can support the liver in its effort to get rid of toxins. Supporting the adrenal gland and improving digestion are also useful strategies for bringing allergies under control. Companies like Biotics Research have developed special products to support the immune system and help bring allergies under control. General supplementation is good, but it is best to have a trained professional help you decide which supplementation is best for you.

Finding and avoiding allergic foods is still a good strategy, even if you are working on the digestion, liver or adrenal gland to completely fix the problem. Short-term allergen avoidance will help to reduce stress on the body and enhance healing.

In his book, *Brain Allergies: The Psychonutrient Connection Including Brain Allergies Today,* Dr. William Philpott has some case histories of patients with mental problems who, by removing food allergens from their diet, experienced great improvement in their psychological symptoms. Many of the patients could tolerate their allergic foods after vitamin supplementation.

Chiropractic and other hands-on therapies are also helpful to allergy sufferers. Improving the function of the nervous system has a direct effect on the immune system. Many patients notice that their allergies improve after beginning treatment. Many chiropractors have patients whose allergies improved simply from chiropractic adjustments. It is not uncommon for a chiropractor to have a patient's allergies improve, even when they are being treated for neck pain or some other seemingly unrelated complaint.

One common allergy is hay fever. It spoils an entire season for many Americans. They spend the spring, fall or both taking antihistamines and feeling drowsy. One very simple thing to do that improves the symptoms of hay fever is to go on a hypoglycemic diet. Simply avoid sugar and refined grains (white rice, white flour), and eat every two hours. Taking about 10,000 units of vitamin A each day for about a week can relieve the itching eyes of hay fever. Don't take large doses of vitamin A for long periods of time; it can be toxic.

Allergies are more common than most people realize. They are effectively treated by a wide variety of approaches. What works for allergies is the same philosophy that works for many other ailments: Treat the person who has the allergy and don't simply treat the allergy.

Avoiding hidden allergens often produces miraculous results. It is not uncommon to take someone with chronic sinusitis, asthma or another chronic problem, remove a food like wheat or dairy from the diet, and have a remarkable improvement in symptoms.

The good results from allergy diets can be potentiated if some negative eating patterns are changed. For example, someone who is allergic to wheat and is used to eating a sandwich for lunch every day will commonly switch to millet or rice bread and still have the sandwich. If that person expands his or her concept of good diet to include more alkaline eating and consumes something like turkey breast wrapped around asparagus stalks, the results are usually better than eating the turkey with some kind of gluten-free bread.

Sometimes the allergy sufferer will cling to other bad habits like alcohol, caffeine, diet soda or sugar. Avoiding chemicals, refined foods and hydrogenated oil are still necessary. This should be obvious, but often an individual will improve so much from giving up wheat or dairy that he or she becomes lax in other areas.

**CHEMICAL EXPOSURE**

Chemical exposure can cause a wide variety of symptoms, including fatigue, headaches, skin problems, digestive problems, recurrent Candidiasis, allergies and even cancer. Some occupations that involve chemical exposure are farmers, hairdressers, photographers, refinery and factory workers, airline employees, truck drivers, auto mechanics, painters, doctors and x-ray technicians.

Just living on Earth gives us a fair amount of chemical exposure. How close do you live to a highway or airport? Air pollution is concentrated in the cities, but exists throughout the country. Farmers use liberal amounts of pesticides on their crops and liberal amounts of antibiotics in their animals. The amount of chemical exposure Americans get is unprecedented in history. Cancers of the liver, kidney and lymphatic system are on the rise. For people who are chronically ill, people who have multiple symptoms, who may be described as "just plain sick," chemical toxicity is often one of their issues.

In the midst of this chemical bath we all are taking are people who suffer from many symptoms; they are like canaries. Coal miners used to take canaries into the mines; if the canary died, the miners knew that there were dangerous gasses present in the mine. In our society we have people who are exposed to the same chemical burden we all are. They, however, suffer with headaches, digestive problems, sensitivity to smoke and perfume, fatigue, muscle pains, joint pains, asthma, eczema, dizziness, back pain, neck pain, edema, PMS and any number of other symptoms because they have trouble handling the chemical burden that we are all exposed to. They are like the canaries in the coal mine; they suffer before anyone else.

In general, when you think of chemical toxicity, you think of liver, but there is more to it than liver function. Some doctors diagnose and treat chemical toxicity with almost unbelievable detail—to the point where you might wonder, "How did he come up with that?" Admittedly, some of the diagnostic techniques seem to be a little out there, but this isn't a discussion about what is or is not a valid diagnostic method. What are interesting are the descriptions of the patients' problems, the model of what might be going on. For example, a patient may be told that he has xenobiotics (specifically pesticides), in the pituitary gland. The treatment will include a homeopathic of the pesticide and pituitary support—not necessarily liver support. In other words, the patient's problem is not that the liver has trouble removing the chemical, but rather the body can't get the chemical to the liver to get rid of it. This is another reason why you want someone trained in nutrition to help you with your health and not just do it yourself.

Chemicals can bother you on a cellular level and the fats you consume can make the situation worse. Trans fats are produced when oil is hydrogenated. The food industry bubbles hydrogen through an oil, making it a sold fat. This makes the food have a longer shelf life and look more appealing. Have you ever made a meal that had a sauce? When it is stored in the refrigerator overnight, the sauce separates into oil and a solid material. This would happen to packaged food if the oil was not hydrogenated. Look at any bottled, creamy salad dressing; with few exceptions, they contain hydrogenated oil. Hydrogenated oils are in a lot of commercial baked goods as well. They are everywhere and you need to avoid them.

Some think that the consumption of trans fats makes it harder for the body to get rid of chemicals. Cell membranes consist of a layer of lipid (fat) between two layers of protein. The theory is that if you eat a lot of trans fats, they become incorporated into your cell membranes. Because the molecules of the trans fats are shaped differently than those of natural fats, chemical toxins will adhere to them more readily. The cells are not only vulnerable to chemicals, but viruses and bacteria as well. One of the very first things someone who gets a lot of colds and infections should do is to get off of hydrogenated oils and start taking the appropriate essential fatty acid. Some folks believe ADD, depression and anxiety as being at least partially caused by eating too many trans fats. Nerve cell membranes have a lot of lipid (fat) and eating trans fats not only affects their function, but also makes them vulnerable to chemicals, viruses and bacteria.

Another theory that is a little out there is that viruses in the brain are a lot more common than we think. These viruses may be responsible for depression, anxiety, Parkinson's disease and other neurological problems. This is only an idea that is being discussed, and not necessarily Gospel.

Usually when we think of chemical toxicity, we think of the liver. Sometimes the liver does become overburdened and can cause symptoms. Women suffering from PMS, for example, often respond to liver support because of the liver's role in eliminating hormones when they are no longer needed by the body. Symptoms such as headaches, mid-back pain, fatigue, arthritis, and even recurrent Candidiasis may be linked to the liver as well. Toxins eliminated in the bile can irritate the digestive tract, making it difficult to get rid of a Candida overgrowth.

The concept of liver congestion has been around for a number of years. An overburdened liver that is not doing a particularly good job can cause an increase in pressure in the venous system. Many think that this increased pressure is the cause of spider veins, varicose veins and hemorrhoids. Another thing that you see in someone who needs liver support is blanching between the shoulder blades. The skin is ruddy, and if you press your hand onto the back, you can see a white handprint for a few seconds.

Other signs that indicate liver problems are pain between the shoulder blades, pain under the bottom of the right rib cage (these can also be from the gall bladder), bizarre or surrealistic dreams, metallic taste in the mouth (also a gall bladder sign), poor tolerance of smoke, perfume or chemical fumes, peeling skin on the heels and tenderness when the middle of the front of the right third rib is pressed.

You need to reduce the amount of chemical exposure that you receive. If you are regularly exposed to chemicals, take steps to minimize your exposure. If your job provides protective clothing, wear it. Make sure that ventilation is adequate. See if there are nontoxic substitutes. Taking trace minerals, vitamin C and other antioxidants may mitigate the damage done by the chemicals. Substances like lipoic acid, dandelion root and milk thistle can help the liver to heal. Talk to your health care provider.

Everyone is always being exposed to chemicals at some level. Air and water pollution exist everywhere on the planet. The problem is compounded by dumping poisons on lawns so they will be pretty and green and by using bug sprays, room deodorizers, certain cleaning agents, and other chemicals. This is chemical exposure that you can control. Tolerate a few more weeds and have an organic lawn, free of herbicides. Make compost and use it instead of chemical fertilizer. There are many companies that sell household products that are chemical free. Buy organically grown food and meats that are raised without the use of antibiotics or steroids. Look at the chemicals in your life and see which ones you can do without.

If smoke, perfume or other chemicals bother you, or if you can't stand to be around new fabrics, in new cars or around building materials, you may have to take more extreme steps in order to feel better. Create a chemical-free sleeping space. Seal off all heating ducts and make sure that the room is heated or cooled only with electricity. Seal all of the windows and the crack under the door. Don't store your clothes in this room. Have no carpeting or synthetic fabrics in the room. A HEPA filter will cut down on indoor air pollution. Use cotton for sheets and window coverings. The chemical-free sleeping area is a rather extreme step, but necessary for many people. Of course, if you get someone to help you find the appropriate nutrient supplementation, chemical sensitivity will be less of a problem.

One thing worth noting: A trace mineral molybdenum (sold as Mo-Zyme by Biotics Research), is a co-factor (a chemical that makes an enzyme work) for the enzymes that help the body to get rid of aldehydes, sulfites and ketones. Molybdenum is an especially good supplement for people who are bothered by smoke and perfume. People who get terrible headaches when they drink wine may be sulfite sensitive and will improve with molybdenum supplementation.

Many treat the liver with extensive detoxi-fication programs or fasts. Detoxification is an ongoing process; your body is always detoxifying. If you want to reduce the toxic burden, you can try to do it all at once, or you can gradually improve the capacity to detoxify while reducing the toxins consumed.

You can simply stop consuming hydrogenated oils, caffeine, alcohol, chemical additives, refined sugar, and refined starch and eat pesticide-free produce. Dark green bitter vegetables are especially good for the liver. Eating foods that are high in sulfur is also good (onions, garlic and cruciferous vegetables). The alkaline ash diet would be especially helpful here, but you do need adequate protein to effectively detoxify.

Toxins are eliminated through the sweat. Exercising hard enough to break a sweat, and spending time in a sauna, are great ways to help you to eliminate toxins. Make sure that you drink plenty of pure water. You can supplement with trace minerals and products that support the liver. Biotics Research makes a product called MCS, which increases the effectiveness of phase II liver detoxification. (One of the ways the liver removes toxins is by binding them to a small, water-soluble molecule enabling it to be eliminated by the kidney. This is phase II detoxification.) Another product, Beta-TCP, helps thin the bile, making it easier to eliminate toxins. Livotrit is general liver support. Get help from someone trained in nutrition. He or she can provide you with much more information than is written here, and can help you put together an effective program.

**HEAVY METALS**

Megadeath and Van Halen don't have anything to do with health (other than their role in causing a little premature hearing loss). Heavy metals such as lead (without the Zeppelin), cadmium and mercury are deadly poisons. Heavy metal poisoning can occur from pesticides, water pipes, fish consumption and pollution. There has been a high incidence of lead poisoning among people rehabbing old buildings because of the lead in old paint.

If you do take down walls or sand walls in a building built before 1970, the paint on those walls has lead in it. It is very common for someone to experience extreme fatigue, depression, pain (like fibromyalgia) or other symptoms after doing a rehab project in an old building. It is not unusual to see someone in the office who has been chronically ill for years, going from doctor to doctor, whose problems began within a year or two of fixing up an old house. If you have had a pregnant woman or a child in the house when construction work was being done, have the child tested. Lead is particularly destructive to developing nervous systems.

Claire Patterson, Ph.D., a geologist at the California Institute of Technology, is of the opinion that we are all subclinically lead poisoned. She postulates that people living today have approximately 1000 times the amount of lead in their bodies as people living 500 years ago. Subclinical lead poisoning is not something most doctors look for when trying to diagnose fatigue.

Cadmium is a heavy metal that is particularly toxic to the immune system. One major source of cadmium is in cigarette smoke. It is also used to harden rubber, so it is found in tires and rubber-backed carpets. Incinerators often release cadmium into the air, since the metal is very volatile.

Mercury poisoning may be another source of fatigue. Many dentists engage in the controversial practice of removing mercury amalgam fillings to treat fatigue and immune system problems. Removing fillings is a big decision, and may not be for everyone. When the fillings wear out and have to be replaced, do not replace them with mercury. Mercury is also found in many large, ocean-going fish. Eating tuna, lobster, swordfish and salmon on a regular basis may cause mercury toxicity in the body.

One thing that mercury toxicity does is to interfere with the body's ability to get rid of heavy metals. The body has some ability to get rid of heavy metals, but if there is a significant mercury load a person can become an accumulator. In other words, the person has trouble detoxing from day-to-day metal exposure. One metal that will accumulate is aluminum, simply because it is the most abundant metal in the earth's crust. Aluminum is found, to some degree, in all of our foods.

Aluminum has been linked to Alzheimer's disease, amyotrophic lateral sclerosis (also called ALS or Lou Geherig's disease) and other neurological problems. You can get excess aluminum from table salt, many antacids and many deodorants. Many health experts discourage people from eating food cooked in aluminum pans.

Detection of heavy metals in the body can be done by testing blood, urine or hair. In general, traditional, Western-trained doctors rely on blood tests to diagnose heavy metal poisoning. The problem is that heavy metals do not stay in circulation for long—they get stored in organs, bone and in the nervous system. Lead has a half-life of six weeks in the blood. This means that if you are exposed to lead, in six weeks only half of it is in circulation, in another six weeks half of that will be present (one-fourth of the original amount). Lead (or other heavy metal) will only show up if the exposure is huge, or if it is recent. Hair analysis is still rather controversial, but it is inexpensive and many physicians claim that it is a good screening tool for heavy metals.

The best way to measure heavy metal burden is a chelation challenge. A chelating agent (a chemical that removes the heavy metal) is given; then the urine is gathered for 24 hours and tested for the amount of metal.

Lead and mercury poisoning are well-described medical entities. In children, high lead levels can lower IQ, cognition and development. High lead levels have also been associated with antisocial behavior, attention-deficit disorder (ADD) and attention-deficit/hyperactivity disorder (ADHD). Mercury poisoning can cause mental disturbances and neurological effects.

Low levels of heavy metals may lead to depression, anxiety, fatigue, digestive problems (including yeast overgrowth), joint pain, high blood pressure, heart disease, kidney disease and a multitude of other symptoms. The metals create oxidative stress, burden the liver and even affect the immune system. Heavy metals decrease absorption of nutrients, replace calcium in bone, and interfere with normal detoxification. Heavy metal toxicity can also cause severe fatigue and poor concentration.

## Where Do We Get Heavy Metal Toxicity?

### *Lead*

- Lead was used in gasoline until the 1970s and is still found in diesel fumes.
- Lead was also present in paint prior to the 1970s. Living in a house built before 1970 can be a source of contamination, especially near wood windows. Opening and closing the painted wooden windows produce lead dust.
- Rehabilitating old houses is a major source of lead toxicity. Many patients have chronic symptoms that began with a rehabilitation project.
- Certain occupations like working in factories where batteries are produced, working with solder,

working near diesel fumes, and so on are associated with lead poisoning.
- Some older homes have lead pipes, and lead is also found in the tap water. Hardware stores now sell kits for testing lead in tap water.
- Because it was prevalent in air pollution prior to 1970, lead is concentrated in the soil in some areas. It has turned up in produce.
- Some hair dyes and eye makeup contain lead.
- Some ceramic dyes contain lead, and food served on a cracked or chipped ceramic plate colored with lead dye may contain lead.
- Some calcium supplements are contaminated with lead, especially those derived from limestone (dolomite).

## *Mercury*

- Dental amalgams are a major source of mercury in the body. This is a controversial subject; however, the controversy does not center on whether or not the mercury is absorbed, but how much mercury contributes to health problems.
- Mercury is found in tuna and other seafood.
- Shark cartilage supplements are a source of mercury.

## *Cadmium*

- Cigarette smoke is a major source of cadmium.
- Workers in certain industries, such as battery production, are exposed to cadmium.
- Cadmium is found in insecticides.

## Finding Heavy Metal Toxicity

*Blood tests:* Children are routinely screened for lead with blood tests. This is a good practice because children are the ones who are most adversely affected by lead toxicity. Developing nervous systems are susceptible to lead. It decreases IQ, is linked to disruptive behavior, ADD and ADHD. It has been argued that blood tests for heavy metals are not entirely effective. The body tends to store heavy metals in the soft tissue, and blood tests are only good to demonstrate recent exposure or when very high levels of the heavy metal are present.

*Hair analysis:* This is useful for finding heavy metals. Very often the presence of heavy metal in hair reflects the soft-tissue burden. Hair analysis is not the most accurate way to measure heavy metal toxicity, but it's a good screening tool. It is hard to tell how much metal is present from a hair analysis, but if metals are found in the hair, they are present in the body. Sometimes people have heavy metal toxicity, but the metal doesn't show in the hair analysis. These are usually the sickest people; they have very poor ability to detoxify themselves from the metal. Hair analysis has received some bad publicity lately because some nutritionists use hair to determine nutritional status and diagnosing health issues like thyroid and adrenal problems—hair analysis is a very poor tool for that. Find a reputable laboratory; avoid labs that sell you supplements or that diagnose endocrine and other health problems based only on the results of a hair analysis. Doctor's Data in West Chicago, Illinois is a good lab for hair analysis.

*Chelation challenge:* One of the most accurate ways to find heavy metals in the body is to take a chelating agent (a drug that binds to heavy metal) and measure the amount of heavy metal found in the urine over the next 24 hours. Unlike a blood test, this method will find metal that is stored in the body. Unlike hair analysis, a chelation challenge gives an idea of how much of the metal is present.

If heavy metals are found, chelation therapy is very effective at eliminating them. In chelation therapy, EDTA (or another chemical, depending on the metal), is injected into the bloodstream. (EDTA is the most commonly used for lead.) The EDTA binds to metals like lead or mercury and enables it to be eliminated from the bloodstream through the kidneys. EDTA also removes some beneficial minerals like magnesium, zinc, calcium, selenium and so on. Mineral supplementation is necessary while undergoing chelation. Another chelating agent, DMSA, has gained popularity because it is available over the counter and can be taken orally.

Chelation, even with oral DMSA, is often unpleasant. Some physicians will use lifestyle changes and nutrients to help reduce the heavy metal burden. Here are some of the things that can be done to get rid of heavy metals:

- *Exercise:* Exercise increases movement, lymphatic drainage, tissue oxygenation and sweating, making the removal of heavy metals by the body much easier than when you are sedentary.
- *Sweat:* Use a sauna on a regular basis. Sweat is one avenue used to eliminate the metal from your body.
- *Eat garlic and cilantro:* Both foods contain substances that bind to heavy metal. Cilantro is specifically useful for getting rid of mercury.
- *Eat plenty of vegetables:* Fiber helps to bind heavy metal and remove it from the GI tract.
- *Drink plenty of water:* Whenever elimination is an issue, water consumption is very important.
- *Eat sulfur-containing foods:* Cabbage, onions, garlic and other pungent foods contain sulfur, which is necessary for detoxification.

Nutrients to help remove heavy metals include the following:

- **Minerals of the same valence as the toxic mineral:** For instance, mercury has a valence of +2, so zinc and magnesium (also +2 valence) are minerals of choice when trying to get mercury out of the system. Mg-Zyme and Zn-Zyme are useful supplements to use as part of a regimen to get mercury out of the body.
- **MSM:** This is methylsulfonylmethane. It is used as a connective tissue supplement. Sulfur compounds are important for helping the liver to remove toxins. Many people get relief from their arthritis symptoms by taking MSM. This product is especially useful for removing lead. (Both sulfur and lead each have a valence of 4.)
- **Glutathione:** This is a tri-peptide consisting of cysteine, glutamine and glycine. It is found in GSH-Plus from Biotics Research. It is a water-soluble antioxidant and is used by the body to eliminate heavy metals and other toxins.
- **Vitamin C:** High doses of vitamin C, up to bowel tolerance, are often useful in helping the body to eliminate heavy metal. Taking vitamin C also helps to increase glutathione levels. Vitamin C has been shown to reduce lead levels.

Other nutrients that you may have heard used for heavy metal removal include N-acetyl cysteine (NAC). NAC is expensive, and some researchers believe it may not be all that effective. Many practitioners prefer to give glutathione or vitamin C instead. If you do chelation, it is very important to take a multimineral. Chelating agents remove good minerals as well as the toxic ones. Some companies make an algae product that binds to heavy metals in the intestine. The algae is eliminated and not absorbed. This is a good product for children. Biotics Research makes a product called Porphyra-Zyme, which is a vegetable extract that some practitioners use to help the body get rid of heavy metal. Products that help the liver to get rid of toxins are also good to this end.

## Carbon Monoxide

In recent years people have become more aware of the dangers of carbon monoxide poisoning. Carbon monoxide detectors have become common. What makes carbon monoxide so dangerous is the fact that it binds to hemoglobin. It has a greater affinity for hemoglobin than oxygen does. It is fairly common knowledge that carbon monoxide poisoning can cause death, literally suffocating its victims. What few people realize is that low-level exposure to it can cause fatigue, dizziness and nausea. There is a simple blood test for the levels of carbon monoxide levels in the blood.

## THYROID

Although controversial, many believe that hypothyroidism is underdiagnosed and that many people who have had blood tests indicating normal thyroid function may actually suffer from hypothyroidism. One possible explanation is that many patients with normal test results are producing some thyroid hormone that isn't active. In other words, there is enough hormone to make the test result appear normal even if the person is actually deficient in active hormone.

One possible explanation for this is the existence of molecules of thyroid hormone that are the mirror image of the active hormone. Compare the active hormone to a left-hand glove and the inactive hormone to a right-hand glove. Only the left glove is useful, but the test counts the total number of gloves, both right and left. If you have a lot of right-hand gloves, the test will show that everything is normal when, in fact, it is not.

Broda Barnes, MD came to the conclusion that many people suffering from chronic illness had underfunctioning thyroids. In his book, *Hypothyroidism, the Unsuspected Illness,* Barnes states that hidden hypothyroidism is responsible for many chronic health problems including heart disease, immune system problems and chronic fatigue. He also felt that laboratory tests miss many cases of hypothyroidism.

Barnes developed a way to screen for hypothyroidism using a basal body temperature. Basal body temperature is taken the very first thing in the morning, before there is any movement or activity. The thyroid is the body's thermostat, controlling metabolism. Body temperature is a reflection of that metabolic activity and people with underfunctioning thyroids tend to have low basal body temperatures. You can record your basal body temperature in the table on the following page. Then, bring it into your health care provider's office for interpretation.

Combining the basal body temperature and information in a health history can provide valuable information about how well the thyroid is functioning. The following symptoms are evidence of poor thyroid function. The more symptoms present, the more likely that there is a thyroid problem.

- Low body temperature. Patient feels cold even when others do not.
- Fatigue.
- Lack of motivation. You're tired, but can get through your workday. Adding any extra activity is

unthinkable. When you have free time, you tend to just rest or watch TV.

- Loss of interest in sex.
- High cholesterol.
- Sadness or crying for no reason. This can include women who have this symptom or experience mood swings at certain times during their menstrual cycle.
- Inability to lose weight.
- Puffiness under the eyes.
- Ankle swelling.
- Depression. Sometimes a patient is on anti-depressant drugs, and what is really needed is thyroid support.
- Frequent colds.

Barnes states in his book that hypothyroidism is very common for a variety of reasons. Iodine deficiency is common, especially in the world's "goiter belts," or areas that are removed from the seashore (like the American Midwest). Adding iodine to salt has virtually eliminated the occurrence of goiters, but Barnes says the additional iodine is not enough to bring the other symptoms of hypothyroidism under control. Other nutrients like vitamin $B_{12}$, carnitine, vitamin A and tyrosine are also necessary for proper thyroid function.

Chemical pollution and heavy metal toxicity can also adversely affect the thyroid. This is one reason why dealing with liver function and improving the body's ability to remove toxins is so important. Nitrites added to packaged meats, certain sulfa drugs given to farm animals and even certain soft plastics used to hold drinks could be a source of chemicals that harm the thyroid. Poor digestion, especially poor protein digestion, may also be a source of this problem. Good protein digestion is needed to get tyrosine, the amino acid precursor to thyroid hormone.

Barnes recommended the use of natural thyroid extract (also called Armor thyroid). He preferred the natural product to the usually prescribed synthetic hormone (called Synthroid) because although Armor thyroid is a drug that is available by prescription only, it is a whole product and contains all the components of thyroid hormone. Synthroid has to be converted by the body to the active hormone. Some patients on Synthroid still have some of their symptoms. These folks improve with supplementation that helps the body convert the hormone. Selenium is such a supplement. Biotics Research makes a product called Meda-stim that contains the nutrients that the body can use to create active hormone. Some patients can improve thyroid function with nutrient supplementation, exercise, dietary changes and addressing some of the other core health issues.

You can use the basal body temperature test to determine a possible problem with the thyroid. Patients take their *axillary* temperature the very first thing in the morning before they get out of bed or even move around. They should even shake down the thermometer the night before (making sure that they use a mercury thermometer, not a digital one).

If the thyroid is functioning properly, the *axillary* temperature (taken in the arm pit) should be between 97.8°F and 98.2°F. Basal body temperature is a useful tool. Patients taking thyroid medication can be screened to see if their temperature is too high from taking too much hormone. You can have a woman take her basal body temperature throughout her cycle and get an idea of estrogen and progesterone levels. If she has excess estrogen, her temperature will be normal at mid-cycle, but begin to drop as she approaches her period and stays low until a few days after her period stops. If she has low progesterone, the temperature will be higher as she approaches her period and will decrease during her period, approaching normal as the period ends.

## Basal Body Temperature Chart

1.  Take your temperature the very first thing in the morning before you move around or get up. Make sure that you use a mercury thermometer and that you shake it down the night before.
2.  Take the temperature in your armpit. Leave the thermometer there for 10 minutes.
3.  Indicate the first day of your menstrual cycle by circling the point.
4.  Indicate the end of your menstrual cycle by placing an "X" through the point.

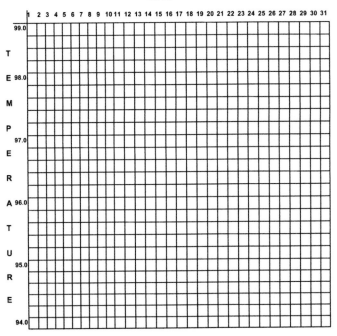

DAY

## Testing for Hypothyroidism

- *Basal body temperature:* See preceding discussion.
- *Symptom profile:* Some doctors will give thyroid support to patients who exhibit some of the following symptoms: fatigue, lack of motivation, weight gain or inability to lose weight, sadness or crying for no reason, lack of motivation, puffiness under the eyes, ankle swelling, depression or frequent colds. This is especially so if the patients have a low basal body temperature. Some doctors will treat the thyroid if these symptoms are present, regardless of what the blood tests show.
- *Achilles tendon reflex:* There is a device that will measure the speed of the Achilles tendon reflex. If the reflex is sluggish, it is an indication of low thyroid function.
- *Tenderness of the Chapman reflex:* The Chapman reflex for the thyroid is at the second intercostal space near the sternum.
- *Tenderness along the costal-sternal joints* (where the ribs meet the breast bone) is an indication of low thyroid function.
- *Laboratory tests:* Thyroid profile. Some laboratories offer an R-$T_3$ test for active hormone.

## Supplements to Help with Thyroid Function

- *Thyrostim:* This product supports both pituitary and thyroid function. It contains copper, manganese, rubidium, selenium, iodine, neonatal pituitary/hypothalmus complex, lactobacillus acidophilus, vitamin A, L-tyrosine, tyrosinase, superoxide dismutase and catalase.
- *Meda-Stim:* This product contains L-tyrosine, glutamic acid, aspartic acid, L-glutathione, sea

kelp, magnesium, riboflavin, selenium, pyridoxine, thiamine, zinc and rubidium.
- *Liquid Iodine:* Contains 75 µg of potassium iodide per drop.
- *GTA:* This product contains 5 mg of thyroid glandular material that is processed to remove thyroxine.

## APPROCHES TO SOME COMMON HEALTH COMPLAINTS

This is not a very complete list of the kinds of complaints that can be addressed with natural health care. In reality, no matter what your health problem, you can address it with natural health care. Even diseases like cancer, held in the exclusive realm of the medical profession, can be addressed with diet and other lifestyle changes in cooperation with the medical treatment. Even if you are taking drugs or have surgery planned, eating healthily and taking supplements can improve your situation.

Many conditions commonly treated with drugs or medical procedures actually improve when treated with natural health care instead of medicine. Traditional medicine's approach to disease is invasive. All drugs have side effects; and when medical doctors treat most chronic health complaints, additional problems are created. Take gastric reflux, for example. Earlier you read the side effects of the drugs used to treat this condition. Any natural health care practitioner can tell you that dietary change and digestive support will permanently improve this condition and do it without side effects.

Medicine excels in treating acute and dangerous health problems. Skilled doctors in an emergency room can keep an asthmatic child from dying from an asthma attack. Their day-to-day management of the disease, however, leaves a lot to be desired. Improving the child's health with diet, chiropractic and lifestyle changes will produce better results than the drugs do. The beauty of natural health care is that it can be done in conjunction with any medical treatment. So if the child does not function well without the drugs, he or she can still make dietary and other changes until it is possible to wean from the drug therapy. Of course you usually can't do this by yourself; it usually takes the cooperation of a chiropractor or nutritionist with a holistically oriented medical doctor.

High blood pressure is another example. If it is dangerously high, drugs will make a stroke less likely. Once again, medicine is good for preventing or dealing with disaster. Addressing the cause of the blood pressure problem may make the drugs unnecessary. A holistic medical doctor can help the patient to wean from the medication as the patient's general health improves.

What follows is by no means a complete list of health problems that can be addressed naturally. Some complex health problems will improve simply by addressing some of the issues that we have already discussed. Chronic fatigue syndrome and fibromyalgia are often a combination of problems with dysbiosis, the adrenal gland, thyroid, heavy metal toxicity and structural issues like cranial faults or subluxations.

## PAIN

NSAIDS (nonsteroidal anti-inflammatory drugs), include drugs like aspirin and ibuprofin, are commonly used to stop pain and inflammation. Painkillers like acetomenophin are used for pain, but are not much use against inflammation. Using drugs to control pain is effective in the short-term.

NSAIDS, however, not only lose their effectiveness with prolonged use, they eventually cause problems. They demineralize bone and weaken cartilage. They actually set the stage for oxidative stress and inflammation; they act to prolong the symptoms that they are being used to treat.

Pain medications deplete glutathione—an important antioxidant and a substance that the liver uses to remove toxins. They irritate the GI lining, increasing intestinal permeability. Increased intestinal permeability creates more oxidative stress and increases inflammation. It also sets the stage for allergies and auto-immune diseases.

Fats and oils play an important role in inflammation. Essential oils are converted to substances called prostaglandins. (Aspirin and other NSAIDS are prostaglandin inhibitors.) Some prostaglandins are pro-inflammatory and some are anti-inflammatory. The type of fats and oils you eat helps determine the the kinds of prostaglandins you produce. Meat and dairy products contain arachadonic acid, which is converted to pro-inflammatory prostaglandidn (called PG2). Flax oil and fish oil are converted to the anti-inflammatory prostaglandin (called PG3). Hydrogenated or partially hydrogenated oils block an enzyme that helps to produce anti-inflammatory prostaglandins. ***hydrogenated oils should be avoided at all costs.*** If the pain is severe, or especially chronic, animal products should be limited or eliminated.

Some herbs are useful for controlling pain. Feverfew does many of the same things that aspirin does. It does one thing effectively that aspirin does not. In many cases, feverfew is effective in treating migraine headaches. Ginger is a good painkiller as is curcumin (an extract of cumin).

Enzymes help to control pain and inflammation. Pancreatic enzymes and vegetable enzymes are most effective for pain control when they are taken on an empty stomach. Biotics Research makes Intenzyme Forte for this purpose. Taken on an empty stomach, some of the enzyme is absorbed intact. The enzyme removes cellular debris associated with inflammation. It sort of cleans house, which reduces pain and inflammation. It is important to take the enzymes on an empty stomach. When taken with food they help your digestion, but not your pain.

Steps you can take to control pain naturally include the following:

- Absolutely avoid hydrogenated oil. Avoid other pro-inflammatory foods like animal products, refined sugar and chemical additives.
- Eat plenty of vegetables.
- Drink plenty of water.
- Take fish oil, flax oil or other essential fatty acid. (Your health care provider can tell which is best for you.)
- Take enzymes on an empty stomach. (Again, a trained professional can help you to determine dosage and frequency.) Enzymes are especially effective for treating acute pain.

Many people are amazed at how well these simple changes work to eliminate pain.

### Additional Help If You Have Been Taking NSAIDS or Other Pain Medication Long-Term

If you have been taking drugs long-term, getting your pain under control is a little trickier. You have to undo the damage done by the drugs. There is also a rebound effect. In other words, symptoms will sometimes flare up when you suddenly stop taking the painkiller. You are not meant to self-medicate for a long time with these products. You may need to speak with a medical practitioner.

One strategy to get off medications is to slowly reduce the amount. Start by extending the time between doses. Drugs that are taken every four hours can often be taken every five or six hours. Extend the time to every eight or nine hours and so on. Do this while you are making the nutritional changes suggested earlier in this section. If the drugs are prescription drugs, discuss dosages with your doctor. Never change his or her recommendations on your own.

Nutritional support will help make the pain medication less necessary, and it will help to undo the damage done by the pain medication. Here are some additional nutritional suggestions:

- Heal the GI lining. These drugs have damaged it. You can take IPS, aloe vera juice, fresh cabbage juice, whey (made from goat's milk), glutamine, bioflavenoids or other substance to heal the intestinal lining.
- You may need to take a general antioxidant. BioProtect from Biotics Research is a good choice.
- You may need to take nutrients to support and heal your liver. Milk thistle, dandelion root, lipoic acid and glutathione are all useful.
- Take glutathione. Medications deplete the body's supply of glutathione.
- Balance the body's structure. Chiropractic and other hands-on techniques are effective in reducing nerve irritation and muscle spasm. In fact, many chiropractors get excellent results in eliminating pain without using any nutritional therapy. Of course, results improve when patients follow the nutritional rules of the Healing Diet. Techniques like craniosacral therapy and acupuncture are also useful for controlling pain.

We are all unique. Any treatment program should be individually tailored for best results. Chronic pain does respond very well to natural therapies.

## HEADACHES

Patients suffering from chronic headaches can sometimes alleviate the problem with some very simple lifestyle changes. It is a better strategy than treating the problem with analgesic drugs.

Taking pain medication on a regular basis actually perpetuates the problem. People who take pain medication to control chronic headaches often trigger a headache when they don't take their medication. In some cases the only cause of the headache is neglecting to take medication; it creates a "rebound" headache.

Taking pain medication undermines the health of the digestive system and liver, and actually makes the problem increasingly chronic. Paying attention to basic health issues, while not solving every health problem, will give good results to most patients, without the side effects of pain medication.

Patients suffering from headaches often don't realize how some of their habits can contribute to their symptoms. With that in mind, let's look at some of the simple, obvious things you can do to treat headaches.

- *Pay attention to blood sugar:* Hypoglycemia (low blood sugar) is one very common cause of headaches. People often notice that the headache comes when meals are delayed, or in the late afternoon before dinner. Some people, however, may not make the connection between blood sugar and headaches. People who skip breakfast, or who eat only refined carbohydrates for breakfast (donut, bagels, white toast etc.) often get headaches later in the day without making the connection between their eating habits and their headaches. Eating a lot of refined sugar (in the form of cookies, ice cream, candy, soda pop etc.) can cause blood sugar swings and contribute to headaches. In general, people suffering with headaches should eat something every 2–3 hours and strictly avoid refined sugar and refined carbohydrates.

- **B vitamin supplementation:** This is somewhat related to the blood sugar issue. People who eat a lot of refined food are generally B vitamin deficient. There have been some studies that have shown that high doses of riboflavin can prevent migraines in some patients.
- **Magnesium supplementation:** Magnesium supplementation is often effective in treating migraines and other types of headaches. It can also give relief to women suffering from menstrual headaches. A woman needing magnesium often has mood swings and/or her breasts become tender at certain times during her cycle.
- **Absolutely avoid chemical additives, especially aspartame (Nutrasweet):** Of course aspartame is a chemical additive, but it is so frequently the cause of headaches that it is worth mentioning separately. Also, people consume a lot of aspartame, and for some strange reason, many people believe it is healthy (go figure). Very commonly people who have frequent headaches consume aspartame (usually in the form of diet sodas) on a regular basis. When aspartame breaks down it releases methanol (commonly called wood alcohol—a neurotoxin). Many people are very sensitive to aspartame. In fact, if there is a mysterious neurological symptom that no one can diagnose, and aspartame is being consumed on a regular basis, it may be the source of the problem. Very often the symptoms do not occur right at the time of consumption; you don't necessarily get the headache right when you consume the aspartame.
- **Be concerned about the kinds of fats and oils you consume:** Strictly avoid hydrogenated and partially hydrogenated oil. These oils interfere with

normal fat metabolism and, among other harmful things, cause the increase of inflammation. In fact, if you suffer from any kind of pain or inflammation, avoid hydrogenated oils; they will make your symptoms worse.

- *Try to be aware of foods that trigger the headache:* Common triggers include caffeine, chocolate, red wine and sharp cheeses. Sometimes the triggers are obvious. Sometimes a food is causing a problem, and it is not obvious (as in the case with hidden food allergies). Your health care provider can help you to identify problem foods.

Obviously, the cause of headaches needs to be found and treated. There are life-threatening causes of headaches, like brain tumors. If the headache is unusual or has additional symptoms like dizziness, nausea or loss of coordination, see your doctor. In general, it is best to rule out serious pathology first. Fortunately, most headaches have simple causes and some of the suggestions listed will help many patients. More often than not, once a traditional medical doctor rules out pathology, drugs are prescribed without looking into the cause any further. Treating general health issues, like blood sugar, fatty acid need and nutrient deficiency can get rid of the symptom by treating the cause.

After pathology has been ruled out and the basic nutritional changes have been implemented, look into other aspects of treatment—especially if you still haven't gotten the desired result. Follow the Healing Diet. Balancing the body's structure, and enabling the nervous system to work optimally with chiropractic and other hands-on techniques, are usually very effective for eliminating the pain of headaches.

Chiropractic patients who get relief from tension headaches but whose headaches keep returning, often respond to nutritional therapy. One common deficiency is essential fatty acids. People who keep getting tension headaches often need essential fatty acids.

Other nutritional issues may need to be addressed. Things like hidden allergies, digestive problems, bowel flora imbalance (like Candida or yeast overgrowth), heavy metal toxicity or chronic sinusitis can all cause headaches.

## ADD/ADHD

ADD is attention deficit disorder. It is characterized by a poor or short attention span and impulsiveness inappropriate for the childn's age, with or without hyperactivity. (With hyperactivity, it is called ADHD.) Hyperactivity is a level of activity and excitement in a child so high that it concerns the parents or caregivers. The diagnosis of ADD usually requires that the child display at least eight of the following symptoms:

- Often fidgets with hands or feet or squirms while sitting (restlessness).
- Has difficulty remaining seated when required to do so.
- Is easily distracted by extraneous stimuli.
- Has difficulty waiting for his or her turn in games or group situations.
- Has difficulty following instructions from others, even if the instructions are understood.
- Has difficulty sustaining attention in tasks or play activities.
- Often shifts from one uncompleted task to another.

- Often talks excessively.
- Often interrupts or intrudes on others.
- Often doesn't seem to listen to what's being said.
- Often loses things necessary for tasks or activities at school or at home.
- Often engages in physically dangerous activities without considering possible consequences.

Diagnosis is based on the number, frequency and severity of symptoms. Of course this "diagnosis" depends on the subjective opinion of the observer. The symptoms are not unique to a child with ADD and a child without ADD may have one or more of the symptoms.

**What is Ritalin?**

Ritalin is methphenidate hydrochloride. It is a central nervous system stimulant used to treat ADD. Side effects of the drug include nervousness and insomnia; hypersensitivity (including skin rash, hives, fever, joint pain, dermatitis,); anorexia; nausea; dizziness; palpitations; headache; dyskinesia; drowsiness; blood pressure and pulse changes, both up and down; angina; cardiac arrhythmia; abdominal pain; and weight loss during prolonged therapy. There have been rare reports of Tourette's syndrome. Toxic psychosis has been reported. Instances of abnormal liver function, isolated cases of cerebral arteritis and/or occlusion; leukopenia and/or anemia; transient depressed mood; a few instances of scalp hair loss have also been reported.

In children, loss of appetite, abdominal pain, weight loss during prolonged therapy, insomnia, and rapid heart rate may occur more frequently; however, any of the other adverse reactions listed above may also occur.

*Suppression of growth has been reported with the long-term use of stimulants in children.* Methylphenidate should not be used for severe depression. Methylphenidals should not be used for the prevention or treatment of normal fatigue states. There is some clinical evidence that methylphenidate may lower the convulsive threshold (that is, increase the likelihood of seizures) in patients with prior history of seizures, with prior EEG abnormalities in absence of seizures, and very rarely, in absence of history of seizures and no prior EEG evidence of seizures. Safe concomitant use of anticonvulsants and methylphenidate has not been established. *In the presence of seizures, the drug should be discontinued.*

Visual disturbances have been encountered in rare cases. Difficulties with accommodation and blurring of vision have been reported. Marked anxiety, tension and agitation are contraindications to methylphenidate hydrochloride, since the drug may aggravate these symptoms.

Clearly the decision to take this drug should not be taken lightly. Unfortunately, many times children are placed on this drug based on their symptoms and without much of a medical examination. There are many reasons for a child to have problems concentrating, and there are even physical reasons for behavioral problems. Before a child is placed on a drug that so drastically affects the nervous system, some of these other health issues should at least be considered.

## What Kind of Physical Exam Was Performed?

Too often a diagnosis of ADD or ADHD is handed down without any physical exam or lab work. We are not even talking about "alternative" medicine here, just good old-fashioned traditional medical diagnosis. A few of the medical problems that can cause a child to have poor concentration are as follows:

- Anemia—Anemia can cause symptoms that may be mistaken for ADD. A simple, inexpensive blood test, called a CBC (complete blood count) should be taken.
- Low thyroid function—A child with an under-functioning thyroid will have symptoms similar to ADD. A simple blood test can rule this out.
- Hypoglycemia—Low blood suger. This is determined with more extensive blood testing.
- Heavy metal toxicity—We have gotten better about screening children for lead. Children are not routinely screened for mercury or cadmium toxicity. Cadmium is found in cigarette smoke.

If a child is labeled with the ADD diagnosis, at the very minimum the doctor should have ruled out the above conditions.

## Learning Disabilities

A child may have problems with reading, and the reading problem may not become evident until fourth or fifth grade. Don't expect teachers or administrators to be well informed about learning disabilities. Our daughter had a reading problem. In the mind of the teachers and administrators everything was fine because her grades were good and her standard test scores were within the normal range. She did, however, become increasingly apprehensive about going to school. The whole thing came to a head in the fourth grade.

Between first and third grades most children learn to read. From fourth grade forward, children read to learn. A dyslexic child will rely on memory to get through school work, and since most students with dyslexia are of above average intelligence, this works for a while. In fourth grade this becomes almost impossible. This is when many students exhibit "symptoms" or behavior problems.

Don't expect the teachers and administrators to be on top of this. Some are, others are not. When my wife and I began to suspect our daughter had a reading problem, the folks in our school system told us that she was fine—her scores said so. Her reading scores were just a little below her grade level. They checked everything but her reading. The school psychologist asked her about our family life; the principal watched her from the back of the room to see if he could notice any behavior problems; and they suggested that she just may be trying to get attention.

She had trouble spatially recognizing letters and organizing them into sounds. In other words, the learning strategy that works for most everyone else does not work for her. When my wife and I discovered how easy it was to diagnose our daughter's learning problem, we were very annoyed with the school system for missing something so obvious. When she was learning to talk, we had a very hard time understanding her. She would omit syllables from words or she would insert her own syllables that didn't belong. We used to joke that we needed my wife to interpret what my daughter was saying.

In preschool she could not rhyme words or tell right from left. In fact, at the age of 10 she had to look at a freckle on her right hand to tell the difference between right and left. This, along with the earlier language problem, were clues to her future reading problem.

In fourth grade she was given practice spelling tests. Not only did she misspell the words, if no one told you, you would have no idea what word she was trying to spell. Usually when a child misspells a word you can tell what that word is. Often when a dyslexic child makes an attempt to spell a word that he or she hasn't memorized, it is very difficult to tell what the word is.

If you suspect a reading problem, you can contact the International Dyslexia Association. It can provide you with information about testing for dyslexia and other learning problems. The association can also help you find a tutor. My wife and I hired a tutor for one day each week. She taught our daughter different learning strategies that were more appropriate for the way her brain worked. Within a year our daughter was a voracious reader.

Children with learning problems may develop behavior problems or simply let their minds wander. They can become poor students, and it is easy for them to get labeled as ADD or ADHD.

**Sensory Integration**

Children with sensory integration problems do not properly process information from the environment. It can lead to unusual, even bizarre behavior. A simple example would be a child having trouble paying attention in class because he is focused on his uncomfortable shoes. It is hard to give a complete picture of sensory integration problems in this short section. To read more about sensory integration, get a copy of *The Out-of-Sync Child* by Carol Stock Kranowitz, M.A. The following information is taken from that book. If you know a child who exhibits strange behavior, buy this book.

A child may be oversensitive or undersensitive to a particular stimulus. Inappropriate processing of touch, movement, body position, sight, sound, smell and taste can all affect the behavior of the child.

### Touch

*Oversensitive:* The child avoids touching. He or she may have a fight-or-flight response to getting dirty, textures of clothes or food, or another person's light touch.

*Undersensitive:* The child may be unaware of pain, temperature, or how things feel. He or she may wallow in mud, paw through toys purposelessly, chew on objects, rub against walls or furniture and bump into people.

### Movement

*Oversensitive:* The child avoids moving or being unexpectedly moved, and may be anxious when tipped off balance. He or she may avoid running, climbing, sliding or swinging. He or she may feel seasick in cars or elevators.

*Undersensitive:* The child may crave fast and spinning movement. The child may move constantly, fidget, enjoy getting into upside-down positions and be a daredevil.

### Body Position

*Oversensitive:* The child may be rigid, tense, stiff and uncoordinated. He or she may avoid playground activities that require good body awareness.

*Undersensitive:* The child may slump or slouch. His or her actions may be clumsy and inaccurate. He or she may bump into objects, stamp feet or twiddle fingers.

## Sight

*Oversensitive:* The child may be overexcited when there is too much to look at and may cover his or her eyes or have poor eye contact. He or she may be inattentive when drawing or doing deskwork, or overreact to bright light. He or she may be hyper-vigilant—on the alert and ever watchful.
*Undersensitive:* The child may touch everything to learn because vision is not sufficiently coordinated. He or she may miss important cues such as facial expressions, gestures, as well as signposts and written directions.

## Sound

*Oversensitive:* The child may cover ears to close out sounds or voices. He or she may complain about noises, such as vacuum cleaners and blenders.
*Undersensitive:* The child may ignore voices and have difficulty following verbal directions. The child may not listen well to his or herself and speak in a booming voice. He or she may want the TV or radio to be loud.

## Smell

*Oversensitive:* The child may object to odors, such as a ripe banana, that other children do not notice.
*Undersensitive:* The child may ignore unpleasant odors like soiled diapers. He or she may sniff food, people or objects.

## Taste

*Oversensitive:* The child may strongly object to certain textures and temperatures of foods. He or she may often gag when eating.

*Undersensitive:* The child may lick or taste inedible objects like clay and toys. He or she may prefer very spicy or very hot foods.

*The Out-of-Sync Child* gives examples of the difficulty the children with the various sensory integration problems have. It explains instances of unusual behavior in school and in play. The book gives drug-free strategies for parents. It helps parents to understand their children and gives them ways to help. If you know any child with a behavior problem, difficulty learning, playing or fitting in, buy this book. You will recognize children that you know by the behavior described in this book.

One thing worth noting: Sensory integration problems have been associated with low serotonin levels. Exercise increases serotonin. There are some doctors who think that we are seeing so much ADD (also possibly a serotonin problem) and sensory integration problems because children spend too much time in front of the TV, computers and video games and not enough time playing.

**Alternative Therapies**

Hypoglycemia, thyroid problems, anemia, learning disabilities and sensory integration problems may all be misdiagnosed as ADD or ADHD. So far, we have only discussed things that should be recognized by a traditional medical doctor (although sensory integration is not yet a recognized diagnosis). The message is that even if you do not believe in alternative therapies, at least do a thorough investigation of the child's problems before resorting to a mind-altering drug. Too often a drug is prescribed after a short interview, with no exam, no lab work and no investigation into the source of the child's problem. You do not have to believe in alternative medicine to know that this is not right. Ritalin may affect the behavior of the learning-disabled fifth grader, but not improve grades. Ritalin may have no effect on the child with a sensory integration problem. Sometimes Prozac or heavier drugs are used—this is sad and unnecessary.

Alternative health care may offer some answers for children diagnosed with ADD or ADHD. Ritalin may offer symptomatic control—but no one knows why it works and it certainly does not address the cause. The idea of holistic care is to treat the patient, not the disease.

## Nutrition

It seems strange to think of nutrition as "alternative care," but many doctors see it that way. It is not uncommon to hear, "Vitamins do not cure disease," from medical doctors. In a sense, they are right. Vitamins do not cure disease, but there is one very important exception. Vitamins cure vitamin deficiency. What constitutes vitamin deficiency is where all the controversy lies.

A recent survey conducted by the National Cancer Institute asked Americans about their diet from the previous day. Only 9% of those asked consumed three or more servings of vegetables or two or more servings of fruit on the previous day. One in nine surveyed had no servings of fruits or vegetables on the previous day.

Clearly, such eating habits create nutrient deficiency. When a diagnosis of ADD or ADHD is handed down it is important to consider the child's diet. Don't think of it in an overly simplistic point of view, "He eats sugar, he gets wired." Think of it as a poor diet creating a health problem.

***Essential fatty acids:*** Packaged food, fried food and junk foods are loaded with hydrogenated oils and partially hydrogenated oils. Cells, especially nerve cells, need oil (fat) for the integrity of the cell membrane. Hydrogenated oils contain trans fats that do not belong in the diet and do not resemble anything in nature. One idea nutritionists have about the cause of ADD is that the trans fats become incorporated into the nerve cells in the brain, making transmission of nerve impulses faulty. The trans fats may also be more permeable to chemical toxins and viruses. The solution is to give the child flax oil or DHA and remove all hydrogenated or partially hydrogenated oil from the diet. Even if the nerve cell theory is not true, this is an excellent suggestion for the health of your child.

**Sugar:** *The New England Journal of Medicine* recently published a flawed study that ostensibly disproved the link between hyperactive children and sugar consumption. This subject needs to be more closely examined. Children who eat a lot of sugar are vitamin deficient—especially in B vitamins and in minerals. A large percentage of their food is starch, which is turned to sugar by the body. Lots of parents think that bagels, English muffins, and sugar-free cereals are healthy. What they need to realize is that starch and sugar are essentially the same thing. Starch and sugar deplete B vitamins, vitamin C and minerals. Sugar also stresses the adrenal glands. Some holistic practitioners think that Ritalin mimics the output of the adrenal gland and if you give up sugar and support the adrenals, you will get a better result.

**B vitamins:** Deficiency in B vitamins causes neurologic symptoms. Traditional medicine only recognizes a thiamine deficiency as beriberi or a niacin deficiency as pellagra. What about subclinical deficiencies? Nervousness, poor concentration, fatigue, depression, poor sleep, forgetfulness and other symptoms can all be caused by not having enough B vitamins. B vitamins are very important for mental function. Eating a lot of sugar and refined carbohydrate depletes B vitamins. One of the most common deficiencies is folic acid. Folic acid is necessary to produce serotonin and norepinephrin (important neurotransmitters, or brain chemicals). Folic acid is found in fresh green produce. How many children get enough green vegetables? We can get a liquid folic acid and a liquid multivitamin that can be placed in juice. Often the results are amazing. Of course nothing replaces a good diet, but that is sometimes difficult to accomplish.

***Chemical additives:*** Read Ruth Winter's book on chemical additives. You will see that many of them cause poor concentration, fatigue and trouble with the nervous system. Aspartame, sold under the brand name Nutrasweet or Equal found in many sugar-free snacks, creates methanol (a neurotoxin) in the body.

***Minerals:*** ADHD has been linked to zinc/copper imbalance. Trace mineral deficiency has been linked to allergies. Minerals are often the cofactors that enable enzymes to work.

***Amino acids:*** Amino acids are the building blocks of protein. A diet high in junk food, poor digestion and vegetarianism can cause a deficiency of certain amino acids. There are lab tests to determine amino acid status.

***Hidden allergies, Candidiasis and heavy metal toxicity:*** If you have gone to a nutritionist or an alternative health practitioner, you may have heard one or all of these terms. *Candida albicans* is a yeast that grows in the intestine. A diet high in sugar or heavy use of antibiotics can cause high levels of *Candida*, which causes nutritional deficiency and toxicity. The chemical toxins from the yeast can cause fatigue, nervousness and poor concentration (among a wide variety of symptoms). Hidden allergies can also be a problem. A favorite food, eaten every day, often is the culprit causing the ADD or ADHD. Great improvement is often achieved by following simple, basic nutritional rules, like those presented earlier in the book.

*Chiropractic:* Of course chiropractors treat ADD and ADHD; the nervous system is involved, isn't it? Many times jamming in the upper cervical spine affects the dura (a membrane covering the brain and spinal cord), affecting the entire nervous system. This can happen from the trauma of birth. Chiropractors treat this, often with great success.

*Craniosacral therapy:* The cranial bones move, much the same way that the gills of a fish move. This movement is vital to the correct function of the central nervous system. Birth trauma, head trauma or jaw dysfunction may interfere with this movement, creating the symptoms of ADD or ADHD. Babies who are born by Cesearean section are often in need of craniosacral therapy. The contractions of the birth canal serve to pump the craniosacral system during birth. Babies born by C-section do not have this benefit. Learn more about craniosacral therapy by going to www.upledger.com.

Many times parents will try nutrition, put their child on a hypoallergenic diet or try some alternative therapy without getting the desired result. Then the parents are frustrated. The point is, *all* of the pertinent issues must be addressed. Giving a child who has a learning disability a dairy- and wheat-free diet may benefit his or her health, but it will not correct the learning disability. You can give vitamins to a child with sensory integration issues and still not solve the problem. By all means, improve the health and nutrition of your child—there's a chance that it will improve the ADD. If not, there may be other issues that need to be addressed. The idea is not to treat ADD or ADHD, but rather treat the patient who has the condition. Don't merely get rid of the symptom, but find the cause and correct it. Health is not merely the absence of disease; health is optimal function.

## ALCOHOLISM

Alcohol is a toxin that damages every organ in your body. It damages the lining of the gastrointestinal tract. It can cause a condition known as leaky gut, which causes things that were never intended to get into the bloodstream to be absorbed from the digestive system. Leaky gut can cause allergies because the immune system works to defend the body against proteins and other materials that are inappropriately absorbed.

Even moderate drinking is a problem if you suffer from fatigue. Alcohol is a toxic burden on your body, and it takes energy to detoxify from drinking.

Nutrition is a much-neglected area in the treatment of alcoholics. Good nutrition and nutritional supplementation can be very helpful to recovering alcoholics.

Because of problems with absorption, poor enzyme function, poor diet and destruction of cells, alcoholics are deficient in just about every nutrient there is. Alcoholics commonly suffer from depression, anxiety, tremors, fatigue and neuropathies. Many of the symptoms are directly due to the toxic effects of the alcohol; many are due to the chronic malnutrition common in alcoholics.

Most standard nutritional texts discuss nutritional deficiencies in terms of the disease states caused by extreme deficiency. Even if a severe disease state does not exist, a slight deficiency may cause slight symptoms. For instance, if an extreme deficiency causes delirium, perhaps a slight deficiency may cause poor concentration.

Read the symptoms of the various vitamin deficiencies, you may notice that they are remarkably similar to the symptoms of alcoholism. Neurological changes, muscle wasting, skin problems, ulcerations, defects in mucous membranes, depression, anxiety, confusion and craving for alcohol are all symptoms associated with alcoholism, but they can be caused by nutrient deficiency.

The symptoms of alcoholism are largely due to the fact that it leads to deficiencies in virtually every vitamin and mineral. It is obvious that these nutrients need to be replaced in the recovering alcoholic. Recovery is so much easier when good nutrition and vitamin supplementation are part of the regimen than it is when good nutrition is ignored.

Deficiency of vitamin A can lead to night blindness, sexual dysfunction, dryness of the eyes, skin problems and problems with the integrity of the mucosa. (Mucosa is the tissue that lines the inside of the nose, mouth and other areas inside of the body.) A lack of vitamin A and zinc can also diminish the sense of taste and smell. An alcoholic who is still drinking, and who supplements with vitamin A, however, will hasten the damage to his or her liver.

A study published in the *British Journal of Addiction*, in 1977, showed that rats deficient in vitamin B complex were more likely to choose alcohol than water. Alcoholics tend to be deficient in vitamin B complex because of poor absorption or an inadequate diet. Thiamine ($B_1$) is water soluble and nontoxic even in very large doses. The disease beriberi is caused by a thiamine deficiency. The symptoms are fatigue, anorexia, weight loss, GI disorders and weakness. The muscles also become tender and atrophied. Another study was published in the *British Journal of Nutrition* in 1980. Rats were given alcohol as their only fluid for one week. The rats also had varying levels of thiamine in their diet. In the following weeks they were allowed to choose between alcohol and water. Rats on a high-thiamine diet (20 mg/kg) drank only one-fifth as much alcohol as rats fed a low-thiamine diet (4 mg/kg). Rats fed a thiamine-deficient diet showed a tendency to increase alcohol drinking when intake was expressed relative to total energy intake.

Wernike's Syndrome, whose sufferers have neurological symptoms varying from mild confusion to coma, may be caused by a thiamine deficiency. If the thiamine deficiency persists, it leads to Korsakoff's psychosis, in which the neurological damage is permanent. Treatment with thiamine has been shown to improve alcoholic neuropathy. In fact, alcoholics who discontinue drinking, but were fed a thiamine-deficient diet had no improvement in their neuropathy. When thiamine was introduced to the diet, all of the subjects improved.

Riboflavin deficiency can lead to bloodshot, itching and burning eyes that are sensitive to light. It can also lead to stomatitis and glossitis—red, smooth tongue and cracks at the corner of the mouth. Deficiency can also lead to skin lesions. Deficiency is rare in isolation, and often exists in conjunction with deficiencies in other B vitamins. Extreme niacin deficiency leads to pellagra, which has symptoms known as the three Ds: dermatitis, diarrhea and dementia. All parts of the digestive tract are affected. The mouth may be severely inflamed. The tongue is swollen, corroded and bright red. Diarrhea may be accompanied by vomiting. The patient may become achlorhydric (completely lacking stomach acid). Achlorhydra will cause widespread vitamin deficiencies due to lack of absorption. The achlorhydra also may lead to intestinal infection. Lack of niacin also leads to nervous system disorders including irritability, headache, insomnia, memory loss and emotional instability. In advanced stages, delirium and catatonia may develop then convulsions, coma and death.

As with the other B vitamins, niacin deficiency doesn't usually exist alone. Also, like other B vitamins, niacin is water soluble and is nontoxic. However, large doses of niacin will produce an unpleasant flushing and itching of the skin. Prolonged and excessive doses may produce liver damage and GI irritation.

Niacin has been used to control alcohol craving. An experimental study, published in 1961, showed that alcoholics in withdrawal noted immediate abolition of almost all physical withdrawal symptoms while intravenously receiving up to 1 gram daily of diphosphopyridine nucleotide (NAD), a form of niacin, for four days. Also, an article written in the *Journal of the American Medical Association* showed that nicotinic acid (the coenzyme form of niacin), reduced mortality from 90% to 14% in a large series of patients who were admitted with severe impairment of consciousness or delirium.

Vitamin $B_6$ deficiency may produce mental confusion, weakness, irritability and nervousness. In alcoholics, there is commonly a functional deficiency due to their inability to convert dietary $B_6$ to the active form, pyridoxyl 5 phosphate, used by the body. This functional deficiency affects the neurotransmitters (chemicals that cause the nervous system to function). $B_6$ deficiency can also lead to low blood sugar and poor glucose tolerance.

Folic acid is one of the most common deficiencies. Anemia, weight loss, apathy, anorexia, dyspnea, sore tongue, headache, palpitations, forgetfulness, paranoia, GI disturbances and diarrhea are all symptoms of folic acid deficiency. Alcohol intake reduces folic acid absorption and increases urinary excretion of folate. The *British Journal of Psychiatry* published a study that demonstrated the connection between low folate levels and depression, although researchers did not find any severity of alcohol dependence and folate levels.

Vitamin $B_{12}$ deficiency symptoms include inflammation of the tongue, degeneration of the spinal cord, loss of appetite, GI disturbances, fatigue, pallor, dizziness, disorientation, numbness, tingling, ataxia, moodiness, confusion, agitation, dimmed vision, delusions, hallucinations and eventually, psychosis. $B_{12}$ is only found in animal products. Vegetarians who consume no $B_{12}$ have an adequate supply, because the vitamin is produced by intestinal microorganisms (microbial synthesis). A healthy digestive tract and normal bowel flora are necessary for vegetarians to produce vitamin $B_{12}$. If they do not have normal bowel flora, they may become deficient. You don't need much $B_{12}$, only a couple of micrograms per day. It's water soluble and nontoxic, even in large amounts. Alcoholics often have trouble with digestion, bowel flora and $B_{12}$ absorption and may need supplementation.

Vitamin C plays an important role in collagen formation. Connective tissue, cartilage and ligaments are made up of collagen. The symptoms of scurvy, the disease associated with vitamin C deficiency, involve connective tissue. The symptoms include anemia, joint tenderness and swelling, poor wound healing, gingivitis and lost teeth. Vitamin C has been shown to improve the body's clearance of alcohol. It is also possible that vitamin C may prevent fatty degeneration of the liver. It is helpful in stimulating the immune system and tissue repair.

Vitamin E protects membranes against free radical damage, helps to prevent tumor growth, and protects vitamin A in the body. A deficiency can affect the reproductive system, the muscular system and the nervous system. Two-thirds of all chronic alcoholics suffer from muscle atrophy. It has been observed that alcoholics suffering from muscle atrophy also have lower serum levels of vitamin E.

Deficiencies in minerals are also present in alcoholics. Magnesium deficiency has been recognized in hospitalized alcoholics. It can lead to heart, kidney and GI disorders, as well as weakness and confusion. Phosphorus deficiency can lead to symptoms similar to delirium tremens. Selenium, when taken with other antioxidants, can protect the liver from damage. Chronic alcohol consumption has been associated with zinc deficiency. Zinc is important in hunderds of enzyme systems, including alcohol dehydrogenase, the enzyme that helps the body to break down alcohol. Zinc is partially responsible for detoxifying the body from alcohol. The more alcohol you drink, the less ability you have to break it down.

Amino acids are the building blocks of protein. The eight essential amino acids are those that the body cannot manufacture for itself. They must be supplied by the diet. They are often deficient in alcoholics. Amino acids are commonly precursors to neurotransmitters, which are chemicals that help the brain and nervous system to function. A precursor is the chemical that is converted into the neurotransmitter. For instance, a block of granite is a precursor to a statue.

A common outcome of essential amino acids deficiency is depression. In fact, many psychotropic drugs mimic amino acids and other vitamin supplements. Drugs have been used more commonly than nutrients to treat depression because drug companies can own patents on drugs, but not on nutrients. In other words, there's a lot less money to be made on nutrient therapy than on drug therapy.

A body abused by alcohol (or any other drug), is like a 1933 Duesenberg that's been left rusting out in a field. Giving up alcohol is like putting in a new set of plugs and some fresh gasoline. It's a very well-made car, and you're amazed to find that it still runs. It may belch smoke and stall at stop signs, but it works.

Good nutrition and vitamin supplementation are like putting a little more effort into restoring the car to make a nice automobile that runs well. It's like giving the car an engine overhaul and a paint job. Alcoholism is an organic disease, and good nutrition is one of the best treatments.

Alcoholics Anonymous has an impressive record for helping people maintain sobriety, but results would improve with an understanding of basic nutrition. Good nutrition will not interfere with a 12-step program. On the contrary, taking time and effort to develop healthy habits will make the whole process easier.

One of the easiest things to do is to take a good quality multiple vitamin. Not all vitamins are created equal, but Biotics Research manufactures a good product. There are other companies that make good quality multiple vitamins. However; many good supplement companies only sell directly to physicians, so if your doctor is familiar with natural health care and nutrition, have him or her order some vitamins from one of these companies.

Multiple vitamins produced by some companies are in a capsule, so there are no binders or tableting agents contained in them. Biotics' multiple vitamin is in a tablet form, but it is tableted with vegetable material and it is easily broken down by the digestive system. A lot of commercially available vitamins are tableted with inert ingredients that interfere with absorption. Products made by Biotics Research, and other quality vitamin companies, are easier to absorb than most vitamins you find in drug stores.

Vitamins are not a substitute for proper diet. Horse manure and a multiple vitamin do not make a healthy body. You need to eat properly. On the other hand, if you eat horse manure without a multiple vitamin, you are probably worse off than if you take vitamins with your horse manure. Even if you do nothing else for yourself, take a good multiple vitamin.

A recovering alcoholic should take extra vitamin B complex with the multiple vitamin. Discuss dosages with your health care provider. The deficiencies of the various B vitamins parallel the symptoms of alcoholism itself. Taking extra vitamin C, zinc and a multiple mineral is also helpful. If any of the deficiency symptoms are present (as listed earlier in this section), more of the vitamin that is lacking should be taken. If skin problems are present, vitamin A and zinc may be of value. If muscle tone and sexual function are problem areas, extra vitamin E may be needed. (No, taking four pounds of vitamin E each day will not turn you into the "love machine." Vitamins are helpful, but they have their limits.)

Get expert advice on which vitamins are the best for you. Every individual is different, and it is difficult to create a one-size-fits-all nutritional regimen.

## Sugar and the Recovering Alcoholic

Hypoglycemia is a big problem for recovering alcoholics because the body responds to alcohol much the same way that it responds to sugar. Many recovering alcoholics substitute sugar for alcohol. Alcohol is absorbed very quickly, just like sugar. It has virtually no food value, just like sugar. It's addictive, just like sugar.

Here are some of the symptoms of hypo-glycemia:

- Depression
- Dizziness
- Fatigue
- Feeling weak and shaky
- Headache

Most recovering alcoholics will easily interpret these symptoms and feel the need for a drink. The symptoms of hypoglycemia are easily—albeit temporarily—relieved by a drink of alcohol.

Consuming sugar, also temporarily relieves hypoglycemia, or low blood sugar. Unfortunately, the consumption of sugar sets up a series of events that eventually bring back the hypoglycemia. When you eat sugar, it is rapidly absorbed, much the same way the alcohol is absorbed. The sugar is absorbed so rapidly, that the body overreacts. Insulin production far outstrips the sugar absorption, creating another hypoglycemic state within a few hours.

After giving up alcohol, many alcoholics develop a sweet tooth. They eat donuts and other sweets. Many consume soda pop at the same rate that they once consumed alcohol. There always seems to be plenty of donuts at AA meetings. Sugar can keep the recovering alcoholic on the same neurological roller coaster as the alcohol. Although it is not as deadly as alcohol, sugar can create a number of health problems as well as make recovery more difficult. It is a safer roller coaster ride of highs and lows than is alcohol consumption, but that doesn't make it a good thing.

Ironically, sugar perpetuates the hypoglycemia that it temporarily relieves. Sugar can also cause changes in bowel pH, causing imbalances in bowel flora. This can lead to problems with nutrient absorption or leaky gut and create allergies. Sugar consumption can also cause deficiencies in vitamin B and vitamin C. It perpetuates many of the health problems caused by years of consuming alcohol.

Eating sugar may seem like a safe indulgence. In many ways it seems that sugar is an acceptable crutch that doesn't threaten your health and well-being the way that alcohol did. Many recovering alcoholics perceive that sugar consumption is making it a little easier to keep from drinking, and it is a safe substitute for alcohol.

Sugar actually makes it more difficult to stop desiring a drink. It causes blood sugar highs and lows. During the lows (that is, a hypoglycemic state), a drink can be awful appealing. The sugar roller coaster is hard on your moods, your resolve and your health. Sugar consumption can also lead to nutrient deficiency and allergies. It makes the battle to stay away from alcohol very difficult. It is a lot like denying someone sleep and trying to get him or her to solve difficult calculus equations.

Sugar cravings can be controlled. Chewing your food thoroughly will help. Eating every two hours and snacking on fruit or nuts between meals usually will eliminate the desire for sugar. Vitamin supplementation and eating a healthier diet will help you to control sugar cravings much easier. Getting healthy makes recovery easier.

## WEIGHT LOSS

This is an area where there is a lot of hype and bad advice. People routinely peddle misinformation to separate you from your hard-earned dollars. They create the illusion that there is a simple, effortless way to do it and all you have to do is send money to get the special exercise machine, energy shake, video set, vitamins or whatever, and you too can be thin and happy.

The type of exercise machine or video routine is not as important as paying attention to good rules about exercising—proper warm-up and cool down, and balancing aerobic and anaerobic activity. You need to know that dieting and limiting the amount of food you eat doesn't work; you actually need to eat enough to ensure that your metabolism doesn't slow down.

If you exercise and follow the Healing Diet, weight loss should be no problem. Of course there are those who will read this and desire to eat more "normally." *Sugar Busters* is a diet that is for the most part "normal," in that you can eat in a restaurant without giving the waiter a lot of special instructions. You can shop in a regular grocery store and get all the food that is necessary. It is mainly designed to get you to produce less insulin. Most Americans who are overweight owe their condition to refined carbohydrates and insulin production. This explains the popularity of the Atkins Diet. It's not a particularly healthy diet, but people lose weight because it reduces insulin production and kills yeast.

Insulin is necessary to remove sugar from the blood and put it into the cells. Few people know that insulin also helps the body to store fat. The average American eats 150 pounds of refined sugar each year and gets 50% of his or her calories from refined carbohydrate. They are forcing themselves to make a lot of insulin and creating a weight problem. *Sugar Busters* forbids foods that have a high glycemic index (that is, cause insulin production). Not only are things like candy, soda pop, cookies and other refined sugar sources forbidden, no refined starch can be eaten. Foods like white rice, refined noodles, and white bread are not allowed. The diet also does not allow you to have white potatoes (although sweet potatoes are allowed). Fruits that are very high in sugar like bananas and raisons are also not allowed. You can eat wheat and rice, but it must be the whole grain. You are better off if you can follow the Healing Diet.

The Healing Diet does not limit total food consumption, except to say that you should eat all three meals and that one plate full of food is enough. Limiting calories is a poor strategy for losing weight. It tends to slow your metabolism down. When you deny your body food, it gets more efficient at getting by with less food. You begin to burn fewer calories. The Nazis kept very accurate records in the concentration camps. The prisoners kept on a starvation diet of less than 800 calories lost only a pound or two each week.

If you want to lose weight, you need to speed up your metabolism. Eat enough food—don't overeat, but don't starve yourself either. Get plenty of good quality protein and exercise.

When you begin an exercise program to lose weight, build an aerobic base like Dr. Maffetone suggests. Aerobic activity means that the muscles are supplied with oxygen directly by the blood. You should not get out of breath; that is a sign that the muscles are working anaerobically. You should be able to converse normally when doing aerobic exercise. Do exercises like walking, biking or swimming. Get your heart rate to 180 minus your age—no more. Do this for a month or two.

You can't stay with aerobic activity indefinitely. You've seen people begin to do easy exercise by walking on a treadmill. They start to watch their diet. They lose weight at first, but eventually plateau. If they stay with the easy aerobic exercise, they can't help but plateau. After time, it is necessary to add anaerobic activity.

During anaerobic activity, you do breathe hard because the normal blood flow cannot supply enough oxygen. Fortunately the muscles have a mechanism to perform during an oxygen-deficit period; otherwise instead of getting out of breath during hard exercise your muscles would just stop working. Read Dr. Phil Maffetone's book *In Fitness and in Health* for more information about balancing aerobic and anaerobic activity.

Remember, follow a program like the one below only after establishing a good aerobic base. Also, it is necessary to back off of doing anaerobic activity. After a month of doing the following workout, go back to simply using a treadmill or exercise bicycle, keeping your heart rate at 180 minus your age. Better yet, get a copy of *In Fitness and in Health* by Dr. Maffetone and learn how to tell if you need aerobic or anaerobic activity. Exercise six days each week for at least 30 minutes. Make sure that you warm up for 10 minutes before and cool down for 10 minutes after working out. Do three days of cardiovascular and three days of weight lifting on alternating days. A sample two-week schedule would look like this:

- <u>Monday</u>: Cardiovascular
- <u>Tuesday</u>: Weights (upper body—bicep, tricep, pectoralis, latissimus dorsi, deltoids)
- <u>Wednesday</u>: Cardiovascular
- <u>Thursday</u>: Weights (lower body—quadraceps, hamstrings, gluteals, abdominals)
- <u>Friday</u>: Cardiovascular
- <u>Saturday</u>: Weights (upper body)
- <u>Sunday</u>: Off
- <u>Monday</u>: Cardiovascular
- <u>Tuesday</u>: Weights (lower body)
- <u>Wednesday</u>: Cardiovascular
- <u>Thursday</u>: Weights (upper body)
- <u>Friday</u>: Cardiovascular
- <u>Saturday</u>: Weights (lower body)
- <u>Sunday</u>: Off

Do interval training during your anaerobic cardiovascular activity. Spend one minute doing the activity at an easy pace, the next minute work a little harder and so on. By the time you get to the fifth or sixth minute, you should be working at near-peak capacity. After that go back to the easy pace of the first minute and do the whole sequence again. Spend about 20 minutes (four cycles) exercising. Spend about five minutes cooling down, do the exercise at an easy pace. To maximize weight loss, do this first thing in the morning and don't eat for at least an hour after exercising.

Increasing muscle mass by working hard on the weight lifting will increase your muscle mass, speeding up your metabolism. Not everyone wishes to bulk up; individual goals will vary. In general, if you lift heavy weights with fewer repetitions, the size of the muscles will increase. If you do not wish to bulk up a lot, do more repetitions with lighter weights. It is better to use free weights rather than machines. Free weights force you to use muscles that stabilize the joint during the exercise, giving you a more balanced workout. Free weights give a much better workout than weight machines.

If you wish to increase your muscle mass do four sets of eight to ten repetitions. Gradually increase the weight with each set so that your first set is relatively easy and you are working very hard on the last set. After doing the last repetition on the last set, you should really feel that you couldn't lift one more thing with that muscle.

Most people, however, do not want to bulk up. A great way to increase strength and endurance without bulking up is the "Body Electric" workouts. "Body Electric" can be seen on a lot of public television stations. Margaret Richard created the series and runs the exercise sessions. She stresses form and gives good advice for preventing injury. She also is a breath of fresh air in the health and fitness field. She doesn't hype herself or pretend to be "THE ANSWER" to everyone's health and weight-loss problems. She will tell you during her workouts that if you want to lose weight, you still need to do cardiovascular exercise and watch your diet. Her thing is muscle tone and strength and she does a very good job at it. You can get her videos online at www.bodyelectrictv.com.

You need to get the advice of your doctor before beginning any exercise program. You need to properly balance aerobic and activity. If you do not seem to be progressing, it may mean that you need anaerobic activity. If you are injuring yourself frequently, or developing problems like tendonitis, you may be doing too much anaerobic activity. Be especially careful about doing too much anaerobic activity. If your adrenal glands are not functioning well, anaerobic activity is just further stress to them (see the section on stress and adrenals) A lot of the recommended programs sold with exercise machines and a lot of the exercise videos recommend too much anaerobic activity. This section exists to give you some general concepts about diet and exercise and how to apply them to your weight-loss program. The recommendations in this book do not take the place of the advice of a health care practitioner who knows you and your physical condition. Doing interval training and lifting heavy weights are not for everyone. Your current physical condition, your cardiovascular health, your age and your weight will have a lot to do with your individual program. You may need to spend more time building an aerobic base or make some other modification in what is written here. Listen to your doctor.

Just understand that foods that trigger insulin release encourage weight gain. Denying yourself adequate food will not effectively help you to lose weight; dieting does not work. You need to balance aerobic and anaerobic activity (think of the program here as an example of how to do this—not necessarily the ideal program for you); read Dr. Maffetone's book, *In Fitness and in Health.* Cardiovascular exercise done in the morning on an empty stomach will enhance your weight loss, and increasing muscle mass increases metabolism (that is, causes you to burn calories faster). Use these facts and the advice from your doctor to put together an effective weight-loss program.

## DEPRESSION

In the 1960s people took hallucinogens to make the world look a little stranger, now they take Prozac to make it look more normal. Although the drugs improve depression for some patients, it is useful to look into why they work and why chemical imbalances exist. Obviously, if a person is a danger to his or herself, the drugs are necessary.

Lifestyle and core health issues have a lot to do with depression. Smoking, drinking alcohol, drug abuse, prescription medications, nutritional deficiencies and even caffeine use can contribute to depression. Eating a lot of refined food is also a major contributing factor. One of the easiest and, often, most effective treatments for depression is to exercise and eat properly. In other words, making the kinds of lifestyle changes we have been talking about throughout the book may well be the key to getting depression under control.

The common medical approach to depression is to take medications that increase the activity of various neurotransmitters. You hear a lot of talk about "chemical imbalance" in the brain. Nutritional approaches can often accomplish the same results as the drug therapy that addresses depression and anxiety. Medication is, of course, necessary if there is a danger of the patient harming him or herself.

The two neurotransmitters on which anti-depressant drugs act are norepinephrine and serotonin. The newer drugs prevent re-uptake (recycling) of the neurotransmitters, keeping them in the synapse longer. Patients who need norepinephrine tend to sleep a lot, cry, stay in bed and can't function. They are tired, and they can't get motivated. Patients needing serotonin tend to be angry or agitated. They don't sleep well. Norepinephrine has the amino

212

acid tryrosine as a base. Vitamins necessary to create norepinephrine from tyrosine include niacin, $B_6$, folic acid, vitamin C and copper. An individual who does not digest protein well (hypochlorhydra, for example), may not be getting enough tyrosine. A highly refined diet will be deficient in the other nutrients.

Serotonin has the amino acid tyrptophan as a base. Poor digestion can be one cause of inadequate tryptophan. Some people supplement with 5 hydroxy tryptophan (5HTP) to help with depression. It is a precursor to serotonin. Niacin, $B_6$, folic acid, vitamin C and copper are also necessary for serotonin production.

One problem with taking antidepressant drugs is the fact the body has ways of dealing with what it might consider to be an excess of a neurotransmitter. The receptors for the neuro-transmitter become less effective, so over time the drugs become less effective. This is one reason the doctors must change dosages and drugs repeatedly.

The point is, if a drug that increases a neurotransmitter (like serotonin or norepinepherine) works, why wasn't there enough of the neuro-transmitter in the first place? Supplementing with amino acids may help; improving digestion may help.

It is worth repeating here that physical activity can help to increase serotonin levels. Regular exercise is often one of the most effective treatments for depression.

Dysbiosis can produce toxins that affect the brain chemistry. Also, unfriendly bacteria or yeast can degrade nutrients, creating deficiencies. People with unhealthy digestive tracts are commonly fatigued and depressed.

Poor thyroid or adrenal function can also cause depression. Adequate tyrosine is necessary for the production of these two hormones. A simple basal body temperature test can tell you if your thyroid is involved.

$B_{12}$ deficiency is one very common cause of depression in older people. Severe deficiency can cause fatigue, confusion and even dementia. Mark Goodman, PhD, has been working with people who have been diagnosed with Alzheimer's disease, but who had intact frontal lobes. He further found that these patients improved when given $B_{12}$, even though they had normal or low-normal blood levels of $B_{12}$.

Many people who are depressed simply are eating too many refined carbohydrates and not enough protein and vegetables.

**ANXIETY**

Anxiety is treated with tranquilizers, which work by activating gamma amino butyric acid (GABA) neurons. GABA is an inhibitory neurotransmitter. When it is in short supply, it creates anxiety.

The Kreb's cycle is a series of chemical reactions that metabolize carbohydrates to turn them into energy. It must be working well to produce GABA. People with poor Krebs cycle performance often eat a lot of carbohydrates, trying to get the energy from them. They often cannot get their sugar cravings under control. One sign of heavy metal toxicity is sugar cravings that do not come under control with reasonable methods. Alpha-ketoglutaric acid from the Kreb's cycle is the precursor for GABA. It needs $B_6$ and niacin as cofactors to be converted to glutamic acid. Glutamic acid needs $B_6$ as a cofactor to be converted to GABA.

Ammonia interferes with the production of GABA. One common cause of too much ammonia is dybiosis; pathologic bacteria and yeast can also produce too much ammonia. Biotin can inhibit yeast and decrease ammonia.

Sometimes a patient with anxiety that's due to poor Krebs cycle activity needs the cofactors for the various steps in the Krebs cycle. These include vitamins $B_1$, $B_2$, $B_3$, $B_5$, manganese and magnesium.

Animal studies have shown that valerian inhibits the uptake and stimulates the release of GABA. Clinical studies have shown it to improve sleeping in test subjects. St. John's Wort has gotten a lot of press. It has been tested in patients suffering from mild depression. The patient usually has to be taking the herb for six weeks before there are any results. It has been proposed that St. John's Wort acts on monoamine oxidase (MAO). It has not been shown to be effective in individuals with severe depression. One interesting sidelight is that St. John's Wort does have some antiviral activity. It does seem to help some patients, but in general it is better to address basic health issues rather than replace a drug with an herb.

Another interesting note is that there may be a viral connection to depression, ADD and Parkinson's disease. Research from Germany has shown antiviral drugs help patients with Parkinson's disease. This is an area that needs more research. One mechanism that has been proposed is that organisms find their way into the body from an unhealthy, permeable intestine. There may be something to this idea. There is now some evidence that heart disease may be caused by a microorganism.

Depression and anxiety are, of course, very complicated subjects. Events from the past may play a role. The body's chemistry may play a role. Thyroid, adrenal or digestive function may be involved. Simply being sedentary can cause depression. Exercise is often a very effective way to get rid of depression. This is one area where you may need the help of more than one professional. Addressing nutrition and lifestyle will enhance the effectiveness of any counseling you may be getting. One very common cause of depression in the elderly is $B_{12}$ deficiency. A deficiency can exist even when the blood levels of $B_{12}$ are normal.

## SINUSES

Air pollution has created an explosion in the number of cases of sinusitis, which is the most common disease in America. There are over 34 million sufferers nationwide.

Sinuses are air pockets within the skull. It is believed that they exist to help control air pressure. Each sinus is connected to the nasal passage by a narrow canal called an ostium. The canals are about the width of a pencil lead. Each ostium is lined with a mucous membrane, which is tissue similar to the lining of the inside of the nose and mouth. The ostea are the connections between the sinuses and the outside.

Air pollution, allergies and smoking can irritate the ostea and cause the mucous membranes lining the canals to swell, closing the ostea. When the ostea are closed, pressure cannot be released from the sinus, creating a stuffy feeling and even sinus headache.

Sinus infections become common because the sinuses frequently become full of mucous and become a breeding ground for bacteria. Often sufferers don't even know they have a sinus infection. They believe that it is a cold that simply won't go away or a series of colds. ("I can't believe that I *caught* six colds last winter.")

One of the secondary symptoms of chronic sinusitis is fatigue. Pressure from the sinuses cause cranial faults. Frequent infections cause the immune system to be overworked, which is very fatiguing. Also, sinusitis is a symptom of other things that have gone wrong with your physiology. It can be the result of allergies, poor diet, poor hydration, or chemical toxicity—all of which can cause fatigue.

You need to keep your sinuses clear and your ostea open. Antibiotics for sinus infections don't address the cause of the problem. It's a lot like having a pile of open garbage and a problem with flies. If you spray insecticide, you'll kill the flies, but they always return, because the garbage is still there and flies like garbage. The spray will eventually wear off and succeeding generations of flies will be more immune to your spray. If you want to be rid of the flies, you have to get rid of the garbage. The same is true if you take antibiotics for your sinus infections. But if your sinuses stay full, you'll keep getting infections. The bacteria will become increasingly resistant to the antibiotics; thus, getting rid of each succeeding infection will become more difficult. You have to clear the mucous from the sinuses.

Another problem with using antibiotics is that in many cases, the problem is caused by yeast or mold. The antibiotics may ultimately make the problem worse.

Sinuses that are full of mucus are not well protected by the immune system. They are warm and moist, and they have plenty of nutrients for microorganisms to feed on. The blood stream and its immune defenses do not reach the material in the packed sinuses. Bacteria grow very easily in them. It's a lot like having a petri dish up your nose.

Repeated bouts of antibiotic therapy for sinusitis can undermine your health. You may develop problems with yeast, allergies, poor digestion and repeated infections. Saline irrigation can reduce pain and swelling in the sinuses and nasal passages. Mix one cup of lukewarm water with _ to _ teaspoon of sea salt and a pinch of baking soda. Use _ cup of the mixture for each nostril. Pour a little of the solution into the palm of one hand. Pinch one nostril shut and sniff the solution into your nose, one nostril at a time. The solution will run out of both nostrils and out of your mouth. This is not a lot of fun, but it will help your sinuses. Finish by blowing your nose. Irrigation is unpleasant, but it will help unplug the ostea and allow the sinuses to drain, reducing pressure and improving resistance to infection.

Nasal sprays produced by drug companies to clear sinuses actually make the problem worse. They open up the ostea, but irritate the membranes, causing the passages to close. This creates a viscous cycle; the more you use the spray, the more your sinuses become plugged. There is, however, a way to make a spray that will not irritate the membranes. Take a drop of glycerine (available in most drugstores, in the cosmetics department), two droppers full of Liquid Iodine (not the antiseptic; this is a nutritional iodine available from Biotics Research) and an ounce or two of water. Put the ingredients into a nasal sprayer (like an old Affrin container). The glycerine helps the solution stay in contact with the ostea. The iodine helps to thin the mucus. This spray is very effective for opening clogged sinuses and it does not irritate the mucus membranes.

Sinuses are often worse in winter when they are exposed to hot, dry, indoor heat. Using a room humidifier will help keep sinuses moist and healthy. Make absolutely certain that you clean the humidifier and change the water twice each week. If you do not clean it, the humidifier may become a breeding ground for mold and you will become much, much worse.

Steam is very helpful to sinusitis sufferers. Long, hot showers, going into a steam bath or simply boiling water and inhaling the vapor through your nose will help the sinuses to drain.

Drinking plenty of water is also important. Sinuses are auxiliary elimination organs. Wastes that cannot get out of your body through the kidney or bowel will seep through mucous membranes. Drinking plenty of water will help you to eliminate waste efficiently, without plugging up your sinuses. You should have eight, eight-ounce glasses of water each day. Many sinus sufferers improve simply by drinking more water.

It would be worth your while to purchase a HEPA filter. HEPA is an acronym for high efficiency particulate arrestor. This is a freestanding air filter that will filter particles as small as 0.1 microns. It will also filter nearly 95% of all particles larger than 0.3 microns. Dust, mold and pollen particles are all larger than 0.3 microns. A HEPA filter will take a lot of the pollution, allergens and particulate matter out of the air, making the air cleaner and less irritating to the sinuses.

If you have forced-air heating, you may consider having the ducts cleaned. You'll be surprised at what comes out of your ductwork. Dust, mold and mites, all of which contribute to sinus problems and allergies, can be removed by cleaning the ducts. This is especially important if you have central air-conditioning. Mold frequently grows in the ducts of buildings with central air-conditioning.

Often a person will catch a cold every fall. The cause of these colds may be the dust and mold in the ductwork. Air-conditioning has been used all summer long. When fall comes, the air-conditioning isn't used, but it is warm enough to keep the windows open and the furnace isn't being used. As soon as it gets cold enough, the heat is turned on, blowing dust and mold through the house. The person who catches a cold every fall may actually have an allergy to dust or mold.

Never sniff mucous back into your nose. Always blow it out. Sniffing plugs the ostea and increases your sinus pressure. Also, if you smoke, quit. Smokers are much more prone to sinus trouble than nonsmokers.

## Nutritional Support and Other Considerations for Sinus (and Other) Infections

A doctor trained in holistic care and nutritional therapy can help you to bring your chronic sinusitis under control. Your doctor will know which therapy is best for you, but it is sometimes helpful for you to know the kinds of things that can be done.

- *Iodine:* Taking iodine helps to thin the mucus. This is liquid nutritional iodine made by Biotics Research—not the antiseptic iodine sold in drugstores. One common nutritional protocol for people with stuffy sinuses or chronic infection is to take a combination of neonatal thymus tissue, vitamin A and iodine.
- *Vitamin A:* Vitamin A is often neglected when choosing immune system support, yet it is one of the most useful nutrients for the immune system. When fighting an infection or when exposed to toxic chemicals, an individual's vitamin A levels decrease. Vitamin A-deficient individuals are much more susceptible to infection than individuals who are not deficient. Adequate vitamin A levels help to protect membranes (like the lining of the sinuses and ostea).
- *IAG:* IAG is another Biotics Research product. It is arabinogalactan powder. Arabinogalactan is an active ingredient in Echinacea. It is a great immune booster, increasing the activity of white blood cells and is very good for helping sufferers of chronic infections to get their symptoms under control. IAG is obtained from larch trees, which yield much more arabinogalactan than Echinacea, enabling you to take a much higher dose of this immune-boosting material.

- *Vitamin C:* Vitamin C is an antioxidant; it is antiviral, and helps to reduce histamine levels and boosts the immune system.
- *Cytozyme-THY:* This is neonatal thymus tissue. It is useful for infections, immune insufficiency, allergies, and other immune problems. Do not use thymus tissue for autoimmune diseases; you may aggravate the symptoms.
- *Allergies:* Sinus sufferers are often allergic to mold or dust. Another consideration is hidden food allergies.

There are many other products for the immune system. We haven't even gotten into a discussion about homeopathics. I have a background in chemistry and the idea of taking something that has a dilution of one part in 10,000 is hard for me to believe. But my wife and I take our children to a homeopath who gets very good results. It makes me feel a little like an atheist at Lourdes. Herbs like astagalus and Echinacea are useful. No one thinks of vitamin $B_{12}$ or folic acid as vitamins for the immune system, but they are necessary for an adequate amount of white blood cells. Folic acid and $B_{12}$ deficiencies can result in shrinkage of the thymus and lymph nodes and impair the ability of white blood cells to engulf and destroy infecting organisms.

Chronic infections other than sinus infections also respond to natural health care. It is a very good idea to use good nutrition and proper supplementation to try to bring this problem under control.

Using antibiotics as the only treatment for repeated infections can cause Candida overgrowth, and it can create resistant strains of bacteria and other problems. Antibiotics are frequently prescribed without testing to see if they are appropriate for the organism causing the infection. Sinus infections, for example, are sometimes caused by yeast. Taking antibiotics can give temporary relief but ultimately make the problem worse.

Diet and immune system support can help to break the cycle of antibiotic treatment and re-infection. There is a tendency to think that the presence of a bacteria or virus leads to infection. Host resistance, of course, has a lot to do with whether a person gets sick or not. Avoiding sugar and hydrogenated oils is especially important.

One supplement that women with repeated bladder infections should take is vitamin A. (Get the help of a practitioner here—too much vitamin A can be toxic.) Vitamin A plays an essential role in maintaining skin and mucus membranes. Repeated infections can make a smooth surface like the mucosa of the bladder very irregular, full of nooks and crannies for bacteria to hide in.

Children who get repeated ear infections often respond to craniosacral or chiropractic care. Our medical doctor (who practices homeopathy) is a genius with home remedies. She had us heat onions for our daughter's ear infection (no oil—just put them in a pan and get them warm). The onions were then wrapped in gauze and held over the ears by a hat with earflaps. Strange as this sounds, it actually worked. We also use homeopathic eardrops that seem to help the pain. I know one chiropractor that puts a few drops of vodka in the child's ear and claims that it is very effective.

Our doctor has shown us a very effective treatment for conjunctivitis (pink eye). Make a tea with fennel and let it cool down. Soak a clean cloth or some gauze with the tea and dab it on the eye. It will usually clear up the problem the same day.

A doctor trained in nutrition and holistic care may address other issues when dealing with a patient suffering with sinus problems or other chronic infections. Remember, he or she is treating the whole person and the cause of the disease, not merely the symptoms. Digestive problems, dysbiosis, and adrenal problems can all be part of the patient's symptom picture.

## ASTHMA

Asthma cases are increasing in the United States. Four to five percent of the U.S. population has asthma. The number of cases has increased 60% over the last 10 years. Deaths from asthma have increased from 0.6 per 100,000 in 1977 to 1.5 per 100,000 in 1991.

There is an important role for doctors using nutritional and other natural therapies to help these patients. Traditional medical therapies focus on opening the airways chemically or controlling the asthma attack once it has already happened. Natural health care can be used to improve the infrastructure of the patient's health and make the traditional therapies less necessary.

There is such a strong connection between asthma and sensitivity to airborne allergens, including dust mites and mold that perhaps the simplest and most effective thing to do for the asthmatic patient is to reduce the allergic burden. The value of reducing the allergic burden is well supported by research and will absolutely not interfere with traditional medical therapy. Use of protective, hypoallergenic coverings on mattresses and pillows is sometimes helpful. Reducing humidity helps to reduce the dust mite population since they do not thrive in a dry environment.

Choosing hardwood or tile floors over carpeting is another good strategy. If possible, create a low-allergen sleeping space. Do not store clothing or papers in the bedroom. If the room has gas, forced-air heating, close the air ducts and use a space heater. Use hypoallergenic coverings on the mattress and pillows. Use a HEPA filter to remove pollutants and airborne allergens.

Some doctors use homeopathic dilutions of offending allergens. Using them is a good strategy if you are allergic to a pet that you want to keep.

Go on a caveman diet. If the food comes in a bottle, box or a can, it should be avoided. Processed foods are a source of unwanted chemicals, many of which can trigger an asthma attack. Avoid sugar and refined white flour.

Taking omega-3 fatty acids is sometimes helpful. Eicosapentaenoic acid from fish oil appears to be a competitive substrate for arachidonic acid and helps reduce inflammation. Hydrogenated and partially hydrogenated oils need to be avoided; they promote inflammation. Too much animal fat can also be pro-inflammatory. This makes the alkaline ash diet look like a good choice. Follow the Healing Diet presented earlier in the book.

Asthma is a disease of oxidative stress. This means that pollutants and allergens can trigger attacks. Certain chemicals that have electrons, which are easily transferred, cause oxidative stress. In the case of allergens, they cause the body to produce stressful chemicals. The electrons from these oxidative stressors act like little chemical bullets. Antioxidants are nutrients that act like little chemical bulletproof vests. Patients who take antioxidants tend to have milder symptoms than those who do not.

Vitamin C is an especially useful antioxidant for asthma patients. Low vitamin C levels are associated with the frequency and the severity of the disease. An adult dosage of 1000–2000 mg/day has been effective in some patients. Your health care provider can help you determine if taking vitamin C is right for you and what your ideal dosage is.

Dietary changes are more important than supplementation. With Americans consuming 150 pounds of refined sugar a year, and 50% of the American diet consisting of refined carbohydrates, vitamin C, antioxidants and trace nutrients are simply not being consumed in adequate quantity to ensure health. Also, eating sugar and refined carbohydrates actually depletes vitamin C, vitamin B and many minerals. A highly refined diet creates oxidative stress and inflammation.

Vitamin C and other antioxidants are contained in produce. Patients should consume dark-colored produce. Plants are high in phytochemicals and antioxidants. Plants produce energy through a process called photosynthesis. Photosynthesis produces a lot of oxidative stress for the plant. To protect itself, the plant produces antioxidants. Quercitin, leutin, billberry and other plant antioxidants (known as flavonoids) are sold as supplements and are valuable for protecting our cells. We can receive the benefits of these plant antioxidants by eating more dark green, orange, and dark purple produce.

Other nutrients can be valuable in bringing asthma symptoms under control. Vitamin $B_{12}$ has been shown to reduce symptoms in asthmatics that are sulfite sensitive. In one study the oxidative action of vitamin $B_{12}$ was able to block a sulfite-induced bronchospasm in four out of five asthmatic children. Another nutrient that is valuable for sulfite-sensitive asthmatics is molybdenum. Taking vitamin $B_6$ has many benefits for asthmatics. Many of the dyes and chemicals in the environment and found in a diet high in processed food are $B_6$ antagonists. In fact, $B_6$ supplementation has been shown to improve symptoms dramatically.

Magnesium is also an important nutrient for keeping asthmatic symptoms under control. Most of the studies with magnesium have to do with it being given intravenously to stop an attack. Logically, if magnesium can stop an asthmatic attack, it is likely that the asthma sufferer is deficient in magnesium. Since magnesium is inexpensive and most Americans are magnesium deficient, supplementation is not un-reasonable. This is a very high-gain, low-risk therapy.

Herbal therapies have been used in treating asthmatics. Some studies have shown that ginkgo biloba has the capacity to open airways. Less conclusively, forskolin extract has been used for asthma.

The same kinds of health issues that apply to most chronic illness apply to asthma. Finding and eliminating hidden food allergies often helps asthmatics. Treating hypochlorhydra and dysbiosis is often of value. Chiropractic adjustments are particularly helpful to asthmatics. Many chiropractors have successfully treated asthmatics simply by adjusting them.

## OTHER HEALTH PROBLEMS

It really would be impossible to cover all of the health issues that can be addressed with natural health care. There are just a few conditions listed to help you change your paradigm, to help you to look outside the medical model of sickness care.

In general, traditional medicine performs best with emergencies. Chronic problems do better when treated naturally.

Drugs treat depression, pain reflux, high blood pressure, high cholesterol, headaches, allergies and other complaints, but at a cost. Drugs have side effects and do not address the cause of these problems.

Getting help from someone trained in natural health care can help you make intelligent choices even if drug therapy is necessary. A good example of this is hormone replacement therapy (HRT). We recently heard about research that links HRT to cancer and heart disease. Natural health practitioners have been providing women with safe alternatives to HRT for years, using things like black cohosh, essential fatty acids, adrenal support, progesterone cream and a variety of other safe, natural therapies. Menopause really shouldn't be considered a disease. If, however, a drug is the treatment of choice, most natural health care practitioners understand that what is usually given to women as hormone replacement therapy are chemicals that are not exactly the same as the hormones that humans naturally produce. They can help these women make more intelligent choices with regard to their drug therapy.

The natural hormones are available, but they are not given. The reason for this is that the natural hormones are not patentable—the drug companies cannot make a profit from them. So they make analogs—chemicals that are foreign to the body and cause side effects. Women who do make the decision to take hormones and who go to natural health practitioners usually know to go to a compounding pharmacist to get the exact same molecules their own bodies have been producing—not some ersatz version created by a drug company chemist. These women are further taught about diet and treating the whole body. It is a much saner approach than taking a synthetic drug to treat the "disease" of menopause.

**NOW WHAT?**

The changes you make in your diet and lifestyle will depend on two things: your general health and how much you are willing to do to improve it. Some who read this may not have many health problems and may just desire to lose a few pounds and to have a little more energy. Others have severe or chronic health problems.

Simply returning to healthy habits and using your mind to focus on having energy will work miracles. If you ever saw the movie *The Karate Kid*, you'll remember that the character played by Ralph

Moccaicio prepared for the tournament at the end of the movie by learning four very basic moves, but he did them flawlessly. The four basic moves to having energy are to get optimum food, air, water and thought.

Consider the two lunches listed earlier in the book. The nutritional difference between them is phenomenal. The lunch with the turkey on whole wheat had six times as much folic acid, and that's only one nutrient. Every day, each decision that you make about your food either moves you toward health or away from it. On a daily basis, eating nutrient-rich, chemical-free food will make a tremendous difference in how you feel. It's simple, like "wax on, wax off," but it works.

Bad diet is engrained in our society to the point where we think of food in a very perverse way ("Add chips and a drink to make a meal.") Our local high school has a McDonalds in it. I have told patients to avoid hydrogenated oils as their only piece of dietary advice and had them return saying, "I can't find anything to eat." Sugar is addictive and many patients have a hard time giving up refined sugar and starch. As a result, some people may have trouble following the Healing Diet. If this is your problem, make one change at a time and set goals to gradually start toward a healthier diet.

Another good strategy is to strictly adopt the Healing Diet for 30 days. If you have someone to help you identify any hidden food sensitivities, avoid those foods for the 30 days. Most people can do anything for 30 days. The change in your health and energy will help you to understand the connection between your habits and how you feel. After the 30 days is over, instead of going back to your old habits follow the diet for six days each week and then give yourself a day off. This works well for most people. Try as hard as you can to follow the program, but be kind to yourself if you do not follow it perfectly.

Also, if you are sedentary, begin to exercise. A good amount would be 30 minutes each day. Give yourself one day off each week.

## CONCLUSION

The goal of health care is to die young as late in life as possible. You want to live a long time, but you want to feel good, even late in life. Your goal is to have a good quality of life. It is very easy to come up with a program that will ensure your physical health. Little controversies notwithstanding, we know what good diet is and the importance of exercise. Whatever your health goal, it is easy to come up with the best possible lifestyle changes to move you toward it. Genetics and permanent injuries can limit results in some cases, but most of the time good health is attainable.

What constitutes quality of life is different for different people. Most of us eat for reasons other than supplying fuel and trace nutrients to make our bodies run optimally. We eat for social reasons; we get together and converse over food that is really bad for us. We eat for convenience; we eat what we can get quickly. We grab sandwiches and burgers and eat them on the run. We eat for comfort and solace. We eat out of habit. Eating to simply fill a biochemical need is not part of most people's reality. Some of the things necessary to eat for ideal health run contrary to our idea of what a meal is. For some, the effort necessary to eat healthily will harm their quality of life. They cannot enjoy themselves if they cannot indulge in some of their favorite dietary indiscretions.

Everyone reacts to this information differently. Some are excited to know how to have more health and energy; others can't get over the fact that they shouldn't eat a lot of pasta. "But I'm Italian—I can't _not_ eat pasta." "I just love French bread." "I'll never give up chocolate." "I just like a beer at the end of the day." To some people giving up dearly loved habits will negatively affect the quality of life. To some eating healthily means sacrifice and never enjoying a meal again. Turning down the slice of cake at a neighbor's house seems unsociable.

I remember seeing a man in his eighties. He was a war hero and had built a very successful business in civilian life. His wife has sent him in because he had just had an operation to open up occluded carotid arteries. She made him come in for some nutritional counseling. I recommended some supplements and gave him dietary advice. He didn't say a word the whole time I talked. When I finished there was a silence that bordered on uncomfortable and he finally said, "Doc, you're telling me that I can't have bacon." I told him yes, that he should give up bacon among other things. He said, "I really like bacon. I'm eighty-four years old; so if I give up bacon I'll live what, an extra two weeks?" He felt improving his diet meant the sacrifice would outweigh the health benefits. To him giving up bacon would give him a lower quality of life than to continue to eat bacon.

I had a patient with AIDS who followed a macrobiotic diet but refused to give up smoking. To him the stress of giving up smoking outweighed the health benefits. The rules of good health don't change, but how we approach the rules do. If you can't give up pasta, for instance, and you don't like your current weight, you have two choices. Give up the pasta (or drastically reduce it), follow the Healing Diet and lose the weight, or eat the pasta and learn to love your body as it is.

No one way of living is right or wrong, but the diet and lifestyle you choose does have consequences. Life is a short ride, choose what will make you happy. If you have chronic health problems like severe fatigue, migraine headaches or asthma you have to decide if your love of your bad habits is worth the suffering. You can change your habits and improve your health—or not.

Of course if a patient can't follow the dietary advice he or she can still be helped. You will notice that various supplements have been mentioned. People who have trouble following the dietary advice can be treated by using more supplements and more hands-on treatments. Some chiropractors have gotten wonderful results with many chronically ill patients without offering a shred of nutritional advice.

Obviously if the patient is not undoing the treatment with poor diet, the treatment is more successful. But the idea is not to be a food Nazi and tell people that they absolutely have to exactly follow a certain program. There is far too much absolutism in natural health care. Do what you can, but if you do not like the results, you will have to try a little harder.

A good health care provider is like a mountain guide. He or she can show you the way to get to the top of the mountain, but cannot carry you up. There are several ways to get to the top of the mountain, some easier than others. Some people will get to the first campsite halfway up the mountain and decide that they like the view from there and go no farther. They may make the rest of the climb later—or not at all.

Find a trained professional to help you to reclaim your health and energy. This book has not even scratched the surface of what is available with natural health care. We haven't gotten into acupuncture or Chinese medicine, Aruvedic medicine, or the various kinds of energy work. There is a lot of information that is not here. Also, the information presented here about health and nutrition is very simple and basic. Think of this book as an introduction to some new ideas.

This book's purpose is to help you to get away from the medical model of sickness care and to begin to consider the possibilities for your own health. It is my sincere wish that this book helps you to begin to improve the quality and length of your life.

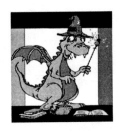

## APPENDIX: RECIPES

Eating a diet that is 80% alkaline may be difficult for some people, not because the food isn't good, but because our habits are so engrained. Many find breaking the habit of eating grains and proteins together difficult. Others may find it difficult to incorporate vegetables into their diet. Often when people are faced with new dietary disciplines, they think in terms of what they cannot do and begin to look at eating as a chore. Frequently they end up with a very boring diet, eating plain foods and having the same things over and over. Here are some menu suggestions that may make this process easier.

Many of these recipes are cooked. You should still try to get plenty of raw food in your diet. There are some salad recipes here so you can add a little variety to your raw food. At the end of this section are some suggestions for fresh vegetable juices. Juicing is a great way to increase the raw foods in your diet and get vitamins, minerals, phytochemicals and enzymes. Regularly drinking fresh vegetable juice will dramatically increase your health and energy.

### Baba Ghanoush

3 large eggplants
3 cloves of garlic, crushed
$\frac{1}{2}$ cup tahinni
juice of 3 lemons

Broil the eggplants until the skin blisters. Peel off the skin or rub it off under cold tap water. Squeeze out as much of the bitter juice as possible and remove the seeds. The idea is to use the white pulpy part of the eggplant. Place the eggplant in a food processor, add the tahanni, lemon juice and the garlic (crushed in a

233

garlic press). Blend everything into a fine puree. You can eat it with cucumber slice

## Hommus

Okay, okay, chickpeas are acidic, but we can offset that with cucumber slices. The tahinni and lemon are considered alkaline.

1 cup chickpeas
juice of 2 lemons
2 cloves of garlic (crushed)
$^1/_2$ cup tahinni

Soak the chickpeas overnight and boil them until tender (about an hour). Place them in a food processor and add the lemon juice and garlic (crushed in a garlic press). Add the tahinni. Puree in a food processor. Eat it with cucumber slices.

## Veggie Burgers

$^1/_3$ cup each of finely chopped red pepper, celery and carrots (you can use a food processor)
2 Tbsp. finely chopped onions
3 black olives, finely chopped
1 egg beaten
2 Tbsp. olive oil
$^1/_4$ cup tomato sauce
1 cup ground, raw sunflower seeds
salt and pepper to taste.

Mix all of the ingredients thoroughly in a bowl. Make into 4 patties and place them in a greased baking dish. Bake at 350 degrees (until brown). Turn patties over and bake another 15 minutes.

## Indonesian Salad

1 Tbsp. peanut oil
$1/4$ cup vinegar
1 tsp. paprika
1 tsp. soy sauce
$1/4$ tsp. cayenne
2 Tbsp. honey
1 cup bean sprouts
2 green onions thinly sliced
1 cucumber thinly sliced
3 thin slices of fresh ginger
$1/2$ cup chopped peanuts

Heat oil, add paprika and ginger—sauté.
Add vinegar, red pepper, honey and soy sauce.
Bring to a boil and allow it to cool. Mix onion, cucumber and bean sprouts in a bowl, toss with dressing. Top with chopped peanuts.

## Lentil Salad

Lentils, on many of the alkaline/acid lists are considered to be alkaline. This can be a very satisfying dish to someone who is limiting grains and other legumes.

1 cup lentils (soak overnight if necessary)
4 Tbsp. of finely chopped parsley
1 tomato, chopped
1 small onion, chopped
salt and pepper

Dressing: $1/4$ cup of olive oil, juice of 2 lemons, 2 cloves of garlic (crushed in a garlic press).

Drain the lentils and boil until they are tender (1-$1^1/_2$ hours). Sauté onion until tender; add tomato. Salt and pepper to taste. Mix the dressing. Add dressing, onion and tomato to lentils. Top with parsley. Mix everything together.

## Mixed Vegetable Salad

Use the same dressing as the lentil salad.

1 bunch of romaine lettuce or two small bunches of Boston bib lettuce—chopped
2 cucumbers—chopped
1 sweet onion (like Walla Walla or Vidalia)—chopped
3 tomatoes—chopped
5 Tbsp. finely chopped parsley
2 Tbsp. finely chopped dill

Toss all ingredients with dressing. Serve. Give the salad a Mexican flavor by replacing the dill with cilantro.

## Salad Dressing #1

2 Tbsp. Dijon mustard
2 tsp. whole wheat flour
$\frac{1}{4}$ cup water
3 Tbsp. vinegar
2 cloves garlic (crushed in a press)
1 Tbsp. honey
$\frac{1}{4}$ cup olive oil

Blend mustard, flour and water in a small saucepan over a low flame. Blend it until it is the consistency of paste. Add remaining ingredients and mix well. Cook and stir constantly until thickened. Allow to cool.

## Salad Dressing #2

$^{1}/_{2}$ cup olive oil
4 Tbsp. vinegar
1 tsp. finely chopped fresh basil
2 tsp. finely chopped oregano
1 clove garlic (crushed in a press)

Combine ingredients.

## Salad Dressing #3

$^{1}/_{2}$ cup peanut oil
2 Tbsp. sesame oil
4 Tbsp. vinegar
2 Tbsp. pineapple juice
$^{1}/_{2}$ tsp. peeled, grated fresh ginger
1 clove garlic (crushed in a press)

Combine ingredients. Try this on a green salad topped with chicken breast. (You can marinate the chicken breast in teriyaki sauce.)

## Salad Dressing # 4

$^{1}/_{2}$ cup plain yogurt
2 Tbsp. honey
1 tsp. vinegar
1 cup finely chopped cucumber
2 Tbsp. minced scallions
Salt and pepper

Mix yogurt, honey, and vinegar in a blender. Place in bowl after blending. Drain cucumbers, squeezing in paper towel to remove water. Mix scallions and cucumber into the dressing.

## Wilted Spinach Salad

1 Tbsp. olive oil
1 cup sliced mushrooms
1 small onion, minced
1 pound of fresh spinach

In a large skillet sauté onions and mushrooms with oil until tender. Add spinach, cover. Heat until the spinach slightly wilts. Toss with Dressing #3. You can add slices of hard-boiled egg for some extra protein.

## Bean Salad

$^1/_2$ cup of olive oil (keep 2 Tbsp. aside)
$^1/_4$ cup balsamic vinegar
3 cloves garlic (crushed in a press)
$^1/_2$ tsp. fresh oregano (chopped fine)
$^1/_2$ tsp. fresh basil (chopped fine)
1 cup chickpeas
1 cup fresh green beans
1cup fresh wax beans
1 large sweet onion (like Walla Walla or Vidalia), diced
2 stalks celery (thinly sliced)

Soak chickpeas overnight and boil until tender. Cut wax beans and green beans into 1-inch pieces. Steam them for 5–10 minutes. Mix oil, vinegar, garlic, basil, oregano in a bowl and pour over the combined beans. Cover and chill overnight in a refrigerator. Next day, top with celery and onions salt and pepper to taste.

## Taboulie

3cups chopped, fresh parsley
$^1/_2$ cup chopped fresh mint
1 small chopped tomato

$^{1}/_{2}$ onion chopped
$^{1}/_{2}$ cup bulgar
juice of 2 lemons
3 Tbsp. olive oil

Combine the ingredients in a bowl. Serve.

## Vegetable Stir Fry

6 large, sliced fresh mushrooms
2 Tbsp. sesame oil
2 cups chopped bok choy
2 cups fresh pea pods
$^{1}/_{2}$ cup sliced water chestnuts
1 cup fresh bean sprouts
$^{1}/_{2}$ cup chicken broth
2 Tbsp. sweet sherry
2 Tbsp. soy sauce
1 Tbsp. arrowroot

Heat oil in wok. Stir-fry mushrooms, bok choy, pea pods, bean sprouts and water chestnuts in hot oil for 2 minutes. Add chicken broth and soy sauce. Cover and cook for 5 minutes. Mix arrowroot into sherry and stir into vegetables. Cook and stir until thickened. Serve at once with brown rice.

## Sautéed Spinach

3 Tbsp. olive oil
1 clove garlic (crushed in a press)
$^{1}/_{4}$ tsp. cayenne pepper
$^{1}/_{2}$ cup pine nuts
$^{1}/_{4}$ cup sesame seeds
1 pound spinach
$^{1}/_{4}$ cup water
juice of $^{1}/_{2}$ lemon

Heat oil in a large skillet; add garlic and cayenne. Add pine nuts and sesame seeds, lightly toast (one or two minutes). Add spinach and water. Cover and heat until spinach wilts (toss occasionally). Place in bowl and squeeze lemon over top.

## Okra

3 Tbsp. olive oil
1 chopped green pepper
2 stalks celery, chopped
1 onion chopped
2 cloves garlic (crushed in a press)
$^3/_4$ cup chicken stock (or water, if not available)
1 cup sliced okra
2 cups chopped, peeled tomatoes
1 cup lima beans
1 tsp. marjoram
$^1/_4$ tsp. cayenne pepper
1 Tbsp. cornstarch dissolved in $^1/_4$ cup white wine

Heat oil in large skillet; add green pepper, onion, celery and garlic. Sauté until soft. Stir in stock, okra, tomatoes and lima beans. Simmer until vegetables are tender (about 20 minutes). Stir in marjoram and cayenne. Stir in cornstarch mixture, stir until thickened. Serve with brown rice.

## Spinach Omelet

One interesting note: duck eggs are considered alkaline.

1 tsp. oil
$^1/_3$ cup chopped onion
3 eggs
2 Tbsp. Dijon mustard
1 cup chopped, fresh spinach
2 Tbsp. grated Parmesan cheese

Sauté the onion in oil until soft (preferably in a nonstick pan). Beat the eggs with the mustard. Add the eggs to the onion and oil. Add the spinach and Parmesan cheese. Cover the pan and cook over low flame, until the eggs cook through. Fold in half and serve.

### Greek-Style Spinach Omelet

Same as above but leave out the mustard; substitute $\frac{1}{2}$ cup of feta cheese in place of the Parmesan.

### Cabbage Soup

Soup is a great way for a busy person to make several healthy meals at once.
2 pounds of pork neck bones
3 quarts of water
1 head of cabbage
3 tomatoes, diced (or two cans of diced tomatoes)
1 can (8 oz) of tomato sauce (not necessary if canned tomatoes are used)
5 coriander seeds
2 beef bullion cubes
2 cloves of garlic (peeled and smashed)

Boil neck bones in water, skim off the scum that rises to the top. Cook until the meat is very tender and begins to fall off of the bones (you can remove the bones with a slotted spoon at this point). Let cool, remove the meat and return the meat to the stock (or not—it just makes it easier if the bones are out of the soup). Add beef bullion, garlic and coriander. Salt and pepper to taste. Chop cabbage and add it with the tomatoes. Cover and let simmer for about 2 hours.

## Chicken Vegetable Soup

3 pounds of chicken
3 quarts of water
2 chicken bouillon cubes
5 stalks of celery, sliced
5 carrots, peeled and sliced
2 cups frozen peas
2 cups sliced, fresh green beans
2 zucchini sliced
(any vegetable you'd care to add)
2 cloves of garlic, smashed
salt and pepper to taste

Boil chicken in water. Skim off the scum, lower heat. (If there are bones on the chicken, you can remove them from the broth.) Let it cool, de-bone the chicken and add the meat to the broth. Add bouillon cube and vegetables. Cover and cook under a low heat for 2 hours. Beef soup can be made the same way, just substitute beef (chuck, neck bones—whatever) and beef bouillon for the chicken.

## Juicing

Juicing is a great way to get vitamins, minerals, phytochemicals and all of the benefits of live or raw food. Drinking fresh vegetable juice on a regular basis helps "alkalize" you. Juicers are inexpensive. They are no fun to clean, but the benefits of the fresh juice far outweigh the inconvenience. Try some of the following combinations.

4 carrots (peeled)
4 stalks of celery
1 bunch of parsley

2 cups spinach
4 carrots (peeled)
4 asparagus spears

4 carrots (peeled)
2 beets (peeled)

1 cup watercress
1 cup parsley
$^1/_4$ cup wheatgrass
4 carrots (peeled)
$^1/_2$ cup chopped fennel

2 kale leaves
1 cup parsley
1 cup spinach
4 carrots (peeled)

5 carrots (peeled)
$^1/_4$ inch slice of ginger root

$^1/_4$ head of cabbage
5 carrots (peeled)
1 cup spinach

Really you can juice any combination of vegetables that appeals to you. There are books with juice recipes available at most health food or bookstores.

1 Think & talk about what you want & how to get it.
2 look for the good
3 seek for the valuable lesson
4 - Feed your mind

optimists
1- they learn more things
2- Try more things
3 persist longer


Karen Angrist
201-767-3764
79 Norma Rd
Harrington Park, NJ
07640